NURTURING BEGINNINGS

GUIDE TO POSTPARTUM CARE FOR DOULAS AND COMMUNITY OUTREACH WORKERS

BY

Debra Pascali-Bonaro, B.Ed, LCCE, BDT/PDT(DONA); Chair International Motherbaby Childbirth Initiative; Director Orgasmic Birth Documentary: Advisory Board Human Rights In Childbirth

And;

Jane Arnold, DNP, CNM, Assistant Professor at Univ. of Illinois at Chicago (UIC) College of Nursing; Currently with Human Resources for Health (HRH) as an educator and midwife in Rwanda

with

Marcia Ringel

TABLE OF CONTENTS

Acknowledgments

N o one person can be an expert in all the multifaceted issues of pregnancy, birth, and postpartum. The knowledge in this manual has been passed down from woman to woman over the ages and shared by our doula colleagues, now friends, who have supported and grown with us, and this project, over the years. Several made special contributions to pertinent chapters and sections of this manual.

Debra met Karen Salt, who wrote "Appreciating Your Clients' Cultural Diversity" (chapter 6), as the Neighborhood Doula Project got under way. Karen ultimately became the president of the Center for Perinatal Research and Family Support, of which Debra was the director. Karen's insights into cultural competence and her dedication to bringing doula work to all cultures, honoring their customs and traditions, became an important chapter in this manual and an important part of Debra's philosophy. In the 15 years since writing the first edition, Karen has furthered her studies and wisdom and is now a Professor of Caribbean Studies at the University of Aberdeen (Scotland) where she teaches courses on race, power, sovereignty, and the environmental inequalities facing marginalized peoples across the planet.

Donna Williams, our invaluable adviser on breastfeeding (chapter 7), was an International Board-Certified Lactation Consultant. She trained doulas for MotherLove, Inc., for 10 years. While no longer a current IBCLC, Donna, along with Opal Horvat, another amazing New Jersey Lactation consultant, updated this chapter. Donna and Opal contributed their knowledge and guidance gained from having worked with many doulas- sharing how to support and encourage breastfeeding mothers through the triumphs and tribulations of the first six weeks with a newborn. Gems from Donna and Opal's knowledge, instilled in many doulas and many mothers in northern New Jersey, will now be yours as they share their years of wisdom on supporting and guiding the breastfeeding family. Their warmth, love, and respect for the breastfeeding relationship is contagious. Many thanks to Donna and Opal for taking the time to transfer knowledge what they have passed on in person, to putting on paper for you.

Carlita Reyes, who wrote "Nurturing Yourself" (chapter 11), began her life as a doula when she trained with the Neighborhood Doula Project in Paterson, New Jersey. Carlita's brilliance shone through immediately and continuously. Her caring and energy revealed issues that inner-city women face every day and devised ways to bring our doulas together to care for each other and ourselves. Carlita's contributions to the Neighborhood Doula Project and to this manual are too numerous to list.

We owe more than we can express to Marcia Ringel, who wrote most of this book and energetically edited our own written contributions and others'. Without her skill and mostly uncompensated time, this manual would not have existed. Marcia's talents as a writer and editor, and her dedication to women's issues, are revealed on every page. She also oversaw the production and the cover design and followed this project through to the final proofreading stage. It was a long haul, but we laughed a lot along the way. Grazie mille!

Adding to and updating this newest version could not have been done without the dedication, guidance and doulaing from friend, colleague and amazing doula, Leah DeCesare. We are most grateful for Leah's updates and doula wisdom that is sprinkled through out. We couldn't have done it without you. In addition, I am always grateful for my Administrative Director, Rachel Connolly Kwock's support.

Interleaved between the chapters of this book are contributions by leaders in the field who permitted us to reprint their previously published work. We have found these pieces to be instructive and moving and wanted very much to share them with you. Thanks to their generosity, we can. In our lives we all have read about certain people, admired them from a distance, and hoped to meet them one day. For us, that category included Penny Simkin, author of "A Day You'll Never forget: The Day You Give Birth to Your First Child" and "The Twelve F's of Postpartum," and Marshall Klaus, M.D., co-author with his research colleague John H. Kennell, M.D., of an essay that follows chapter 10, called "Caring for the Parents of a Stillborn or an Infant Who Dies." Penny's, Marshall's and John's work and writing educated and inspired Debra in her earliest days as a doula. She was fortunate to meet them in 1992. It has been an honor to work with them for DONA International over the last 20 years. Affectionately called Penny by all who know and love her, Penny Simkin brings her natural warmth and compassion to her childbirth education and doula work. She has enriched many of the old views of pregnancy, birth, and parenting. Penny's insights into the significance of birth, has changed the way laboring women are treated around the world.

Dr. Klaus's and Kennell's research into parent-infant bonding has changed the way the world views the abilities of the just-born infant. Penny, Marshall, Phyllis and Dr. Kennell have moved (and continue to move) doula care from an effort to a fixture of the medical literature and a well-respected part of maternity care in America and around the world. Their contributions to this manual go well beyond the pieces they have granted us permission to reprint. Their words, encouragement, and guidance are ever-present in our daily doula work.

William Sears, M.D., graciously granted us permission to reprint his charming 'Ten Commandments of the Postpartum Mother." How we wish these commandments could all come true! As a father and pediatrician, Dr. Sears has written many books and articles that provide easy reading and understanding of the many day-to-day issues to help women care for themselves, their babies, and their families. His advice given in a caring, gentle way, allowing each parent to follow her or his own instincts in parenting. We hope you enjoy his work as much as we do.

Cathy Romeo, who has taught widely and written sensitively about grief and mourning, granted us permission to reproduce two important pieces on the subject. They follow chapter 10, "Unexpected Outcomes." Thank you, Cathy.

The poems scattered freely throughout this manual are by Maureen Cannon, who is no longer with us. She was a septuagenarian. powerhouse and multiple poetry contest prizewinner (and judge) who has been publishing light verse in major magazines and newspapers for over 40 years. She shares her children and grandchildren with us in her poems.

We want to thank the women whose technical talents brought our thoughts and words to visual form. Thanks to Kayti Lathrop, whose creative energy was flowing at the end of her pregnancy when she painted the extraordinary picture that she has generously allowed us to use on our cover. Kayti's insight to her pregnancy and birth abounds in her art. Thanks too to Jennifer Vana for her beautiful drawing in the breastfeeding chapter.

We appreciate the willingness of the MotherLove, Inc., doulas Billee, Melo, and Pamela to share their wisdom and their stories with us and for you. Their support of each other as doulas and of this project has been very special.

Doula work is work of the heart. The rewards are enormous. As a business, doula work does not bring riches. We earn just enough to sustain ourselves. The richness of relationships and life that it brings, however, is worth much more than any amount of money. All involved with the project have given of themselves lovingly and without question. They donated their time and talents far beyond our ability to compensate them financially.

Thank you everyone.

> Debra and Jane

Debra adds:

I would like to extend special thanks to my husband and sons, who have encouraged and supported me in all my doula work and especially on this project. Their belief in me, and in what I do, enables me to maintain my focus and to continue with this rewarding work.

Jane adds:

Many thanks to Michael Seitzinger, M.D., an obstetrician and dear friend who first gave me the idea of going out into the hills of New Mexico to provide postpartum home care to new mothers. Those experiences shaped my life and work from the first day.

About this book:
A note from the authors

Without realizing it, Jane and I began to write Nurturing Beginnings years ago as we individually collected published resources to use in our training sessions for postpartum doulas. Over the years, the piles of paper grew until they carpeted and engulfed our offices. Eventually we knew we had enough to create a book. The dream of creating an official training manual for bringing more doulas into practice took many years to come true. You are holding it in your hands.

The purpose of this manual is to provide you with an understanding of the core elements of postpartum doula care. We hope to prepare you to work with women and their families as you "mother the mother" after birth.

In more than a two decades of training doulas, we have received countless telephone calls from women all over the world who wanted to become doulas. The manual is just the starting point for many issues to explore. If we can't meet you in person, we hope to meet you online, where we will guide you to personalize and add your own modules to this manual according to your interests, experience, and abilities.

Our goal for this book is to provide the foundation for you to begin or supplement your journey as a postpartum doula. We know from the work of Dr. Marshall Klaus and Dr. John Kennell that when a doula nurtures a woman at birth, the mother nurtures her baby. As doulas, we throw a pebble into a pond. With each day the rings that are formed grow and grow, encircling more and more women and their families. We hope this book will be the start of such a ripple effect for you.

Our intertwined doula histories and how they led to this book

Note from Debra Pascali-Bonaro

I began my doula work before I knew the word "doula." As a childbirth educator in 1986, I attended my first birth with a couple from one of my childbirth classes and immediately knew that this was what I wanted to do with my life. As the mother of three, I felt that it would be an honor to nurture women and their partners at such a critical time. My next step was to offer breast feeding encouragement and mother-to-mother support. Soon several couples asked me to help them with their journey into parenthood. I didn't have a training for the care I provided; I thought of it as an extension of my childbirth education classes. In 1987 : I read an article in Mothering magazine about Doula, Inc ∴, of Rhode Island. As I read the description of a doula, I said to myself, "I am a doula." It was a magical moment. I called the organization and spoke with someone who knew of a woman named Jane Arnold in Westchester County, New York, across the Hudson River from my New Jersey home, who was running a doula service called Mom Service, Inc. I soon had Jane's brochure in hand and called her. I was pleased to learn more about doulas, what they do, and how to run a doula service.

Jane became my mentor. As the mother of four, running her own company, she helped me to begin MotherLove, Inc., and to learn and grow as a doula. In those early days, no one knew what a doula was, friends called us "granola and oatmeal women." Hospitals and medical providers wouldn't even return phone calls. On many days when I was ready to give up, Jane helped me regain the vision of a doula every woman who wants one. She kept me focused on the work we had done and what lay ahead, reminding me that change is a long, slow process, but well worth the effort. Jane was a single mother who wanted to become a midwife to serve women and bring doulas to all women in her practice. She returned to nursing school soon after we met. I greatly admired her determination to achieve her goals. Her example kept me focused on mine: to bring doula care into mainstream medical care.

I grew interested in the role and history of doula care and maternity care around the world. I reached to anyone who knew how different cultures or countries cared for women around the time of birth. I talked with anyone who would listen about doulas and the importance of caring for women and children.

Jane completed nursing school and began practicing as a registered nurse at North Central Bronx Hospital in New York City. Although we had less time to speak on the telephone, she kept encouraging me to carry the doula torch. Jane went on to midwifery school through the Frontier School of Midwifery-in Kentucky, and was soon a certified nurse-midwife (CNM) working at the Morris Heights birthing Center in the South Bronx. One day in 1994, Jane called to say she had been awarded a grant from the Robin Hood Foundation the Aaron Diamond Foundation to begin a doula training program, to be called the Morris Heights doula Program, in the Bronx. To my delight, Jane invited me to participate. I will never forget the first day I drove to the Bronx, a community not far from my own geographically, yet so very different from my comfortable suburb. I felt excited, nervous about not knowing what to expect, and keen interest in how this ethnically diverse community would react.

The training was exhilarating. To hear women from many cultural backgrounds share their stories to share their visions and hopes for nurturing support for pregnant and birthing women justified the days I had spent learning and planning. I knew then that Jane and I were right: Women everywhere would embrace this concept. We would work hard to return caring, education, and nurturing to communities everywhere. The Morris Heights Doula Program reignited my passion and determination to bring doula care to all women who wanted it.

In 1992 I attended the first meeting of Doulas of North America (DONA) in Boston and found myself a member of its first board as chair of public relations. I was to work with Penny Simkin, Dr. Marshall Klaus, Dr. John Kennell, Phyllis Klaus, Annie Kennedy and many other wonderful people. My horizons continued to broaden and my views expanded.

In 1994 I was invited to speak at the White House to the Task Force on Health Care Reform about doula care. A few years before, I had been unable to get a local obstetrician to speak with me. Now Hillary Clinton wanted to know more about doulas and the role we could play in rebuilding our families and communities.

In 1995, as a board member of the Northern New Jersey Maternal Child Health Consortium, I had an opportunity to participate in the development of a grant proposal to provide doula care to women in treatment from substance abuse and alcohol addiction in Paterson, New Jersey. The Neighborhood

Doula Project was founded with a grant from the Robert Wood Johnson Foundation of Princeton, New Jersey, and later Healthy Mothers, Healthy Babies of Paterson. Again Jane provided guidance and wisdom as we brought doula care to a community burdened with difficult issues. In 1995 Paterson was a city with a community that was 44% black, 32% hispanic, and 24% white. Unemployment was rampant. More than 30% of the homes with children had only one parent. High rates of violence and child abuse and widespread distrustfulness cried out for emotional and spiritual nurturing. I trusted my heart that doula skills were needed here. One cold winter morning in Paterson, after a month of training, five talented black women spoke passionately of the need to reduce the high rate of black infant mortality in their communities. They vowed to help raise the low rates of breastfeeding, to lower the incidence of postpartum depression, and to reduce ever-increasing rates of child abuse and neglect. They proclaimed their determination to assist teenage mothers, to help women stay off drugs while pregnant, and to prevent child abuse. Hearing my words echoed in theirs, I felt fiercely proud of them. If training and education no longer come automatically from one's actual mother, sisters and friends, they can come from surrogate mothers ... from doulas.

The Paterson doulas had told me that black women didn't always take advantage of the social and medical services available. If they could be helped to feel safe and emotionally supported through the intimidating maze of services during pregnancy, they would seek medical care earlier in pregnancy and more regularly throughout it. Health care practitioners would be able to identify and resolve many problems sooner, so that these women's babies would be more likely to live and thrive.

The women of Paterson and I overcame cultural barriers for a mutual cause. Together, we gave their community the vital gifts of caring, nurturing, and education. Directing the Neighborhood Doula Project enriched my life in ways I had never anticipated. I learned so much from the doulas and the women we served. Running this program reinforced my belief that caring for pregnant, birthing, and parenting women and their families is necessary if we are to provide the next generation with the love and family values we hear thrown around in political speeches.

In 1996, with a grant from the New York State Department of Health, Jane was hired by the Department of Obstetrics, Gynecology, and Reproductive Medicine at the State University of New York at Stony Brook, to begin a midwifery practice there. As Director of Midwifery, and with the help of other key nursing personnel within Women and Children's Hospital at Stony Brook, she prepared to bring doulas to the surrounding community. In 1998, Jane and I began to train doulas at Stony Brook. Jane and I, and the Midwifery Practice and School of Nursing at Stony Brook, are honored that our work to return education, caring, nurturing, and high-quality medical care through midwives and doulas into communities was featured in "Indivisible," a national documentary funded by the Pew Charitable Trusts.

Our journey has continued to include bringing Midwives and Doulas together in North Carolina and Botswana, Africa. We don't know the next place we will be together, yet, Jane will always be in my heart as I pass along the warmth and wisdom she greeted me with years ago. I now train, speak, consult, and design doula programs for hospitals, medical providers, and doulas globally. Doula programs are regularly being started in new communities around the world. Jane and I continue working together to bring doulas and doula training to all women and all communities. This book represents the next step on our journey to broaden the doula concept.

Wherever the doula heart and spirit live, the interrupted tradition of woman-to-woman, mother-to-mother care resumes and prevails. I thank all the doulas who have joined me on this journey, enriching doulas with their shared stories. They bring their dedication and love to the homes of grateful families every day.

Debra Pascali-Bonaro
River Vale, New Jersey

Join me in my weekly e-news as my journey continues, together we are transforming maternity care.

Note from Jane Arnold

Between 1973 and 1978, while living with my husband in New York City, I gave birth to four children. I am from Iowa and knew few people in Manhattan. My mother died when I was pregnant with my daughter, who is my youngest child. My husband's parents were quite old and lived in Florida. After the children were born, I felt isolated and alone even though the births had been easy and uncomplicated.

In 1980, our family of six moved to Santa Fe, New Mexico. I had a hunger to know whether other mothers felt the same sense of aloneness after giving birth. I decided to find out by working as a postpartum home care worker. I advertised, saying that I would do anything women needed in their homes after giving birth: cooking, laundry, errands, breastfeeding support, and newborn care.

My first client lived up in the hills. Her husband was a traveling salesman who went back on the road five days after the birth. On the first day, a snowy January day in 1981, I parked my car at the bottom of her hill and walked up to her house. No neighbors lived as far as the eye could see. As I worked, she followed me around, carrying the baby in her arms, asking me about breastfeeding, the changes her body was going through, her loneliness and sadness regarding her husbands absence, and much more. I had my answer! She felt just as I had. My sadness and isolation began to heal.

A neighbor of mine in Santa Fe was an obstetrician who was building a birth center. I thought to myself, "How are women going to give birth and be discharged within 12 to 24 hours without support and nurturing in the early postpartum time?" Soon I started my own business, which I called Mom Service, Inc. As far as I know, it was the very first postpartum and labor support service in the country. I served as the director of that service until 1986, when I entered nursing school with a plan to become a nurse-midwife.

I was now in my mid-forties, a single parent with four children. I had always wanted to be a nurse, but I had grown up in the 1950s, when good Iowa women married hardy farmers and stayed at home to raise crops and children. Nursing was not an option my parents would tolerate. I escaped into teaching, which was acceptable to my parents.

In 1986, I decided that if I didn't go to nursing school right away, I never would. I pursued that goal and received my Bachelor of Science in Nursing (BSN) degree from Columbia University in 1988. In 1990, the year my oldest son started college, I became a certified nurse-midwife (CNM) and graduated from the Frontier School of Midwifery in Hyden, Kentucky just in time.

In some essential way, I have always been a doula and a midwife. To combine the two in the service of women and babies is one of my greatest joys.

Jane Arnold
Stony Brook, New York
November 1999

CONTRIBUTORS:

Opal Horvat, BA, IBCLC,

One of the original postpartum doulas, Opal has many decades of experience with hands on assistance in getting mothers on the path to successful breastfeeding. As well as a former postpartum doula, she has worked as a Lactation Consultant for the WIC Program, training and supervising peer counselors and helping thousands of mothers and babies for twenty years. She has also been a LLL member for 25 years and has breastfed her two sons. Currently she is in private practice and does home visits in Bergen, Hudson, Passaic, and Essex counties in NE New Jersey

Donna Williams, MA

With decades of experience as a mother of four and now grandmother, too, Donna was an IBCLC, LLL, WIC LC, doula trainer, and in private practice. Inspired by the online learning potential of the first edition of Nurturing Beginnings, she changed careers and taught technology in an elementary school. She is intrigued to combine these two passions to assist postpartum doulas.

Dr. Karen Salt

She is a professor of Caribbean studies at the University of Aberdeen (Scotland) where she teaches courses on race, power, sovereignty, and the environmental inequalities facing marginalized peoples across the planet. She has a keen interest in island eco-aesthetics and the ways that island peoples try to live in balance with and respond to their natural world. She began her journey in women's health teaching childbirth classes before training as a doula. From her days running her own company offering childbirth education and doula services to teens and families receiving AFDC (Aid to Families with Dependent Children) and TANF (Temporary Assistance to Needy Families) to her many duties within national organizations working on midwifery, childbirth, and mother-baby issues, Karen has focused on ameliorating health inequalities, improving women's access to care, and emphasizing the importance of cultural practices within pregnancy, childbirth, and the weeks to months during the postpartum period. She is the author of *Baby Tips for New Moms: Breastfeeding* (Perseus), *Pregnancy Tips for Moms to Be* (Perseus), and *A Doula's Guide to Pregnancy, Childbirth, and Motherhood: Wisdom and Advice From a Doula* (Da Capo), *A Holistic Guide to Embracing Pregnancy, Childbirth, and Motherhood* (Da Capo). Karen has written articles for *Midwifery Today*, *Childbirth Instructor*, the *Journal of Perinatal Education*, and other publications.

Leah DeCesare

Leah DeCesare, who's primary role is as mother of three, is a certified birth and postpartum doula, childbirth educator and lactation counselor. She is also a writer, working on her first novel as well as parenting books. Her professional experience is in birth and babies (early parenting), while her current parenting adventures revolve around kids school-aged through teenagers creating the basis for her Mother's Circle parenting blog. Leah blogs at Mother's Circle where she shares perspectives on parenting, from pregnancy through teens. Leah has written articles for publication in the International Doula, DONA International's professional journal as well as local publications and online outlets. Leah is the co-founder of Doulas of Rhode Island, Past Northeast Regional Director for DONA International, past Rhode Island State Representative for DONA International and locally, she volunteers with Families First Rhode Island as a mentor to new mothers struggling with postpartum mood disorders. She also volunteers with Kappa Kappa Gamma, her church and her kids' schools.

Rachel Connolly Kwock

Rachel Connolly Kwock is Administrative Director and Creative Content Editor to Debra Pascali-Bonaro as well as a Birth Doula in New Jersey and a Birth Media Advocate.

An invitation to you, the reader

Dear Reader,

Women have traditionally learned through story telling. As doulas, we pass along mother-to-mother (and mother-to-doula and doula-to-mother) stories and information to keep the ripples flowing outward.

Following that tradition, this manual uses stories as a learning tool. We encourage you to write down your thoughts as you explore what it means to be a doula. Please consider sending us your best stories. Some may be used in future editions, so unless you state that your note is private, we will assume that it may be shared in print (no names will be used).

We also welcome your feedback on this manual. How are you using it? Is it helpful? Can you suggest good doula resources for future editions? We would welcome great doula recipes, too.

If you have access to e-mail, please send your doula stories, feedback, recommended resources, recipes, or other comments to: debrapascalibonaro@gmail.com

Thanks so much!

Warm regards,

Debra, Jane and Marcia

INTRODUCTION

The ancient, emerging field of doula care

This is a book about empowerment and being in the service of others. It will empower you to achieve the respected status of a paraprofessional in the health field and coincidentally learn a great deal about yourself. What you learn will, in turn, empower the women you serve.

Women who are supported and encouraged to grow during pregnancy and delivery can achieve remarkable spiritual, mental, and physical growth. Women need other women at this highly significant, deeply emotional, confusingly physical, eternally memorable time. They want women to hear their private fears and concerns, provide information they're desperately hungry for, and share their own experience. They benefit from the presence of someone who facilitates getting in touch with their inner sense of trust and faith in their bodies. Doulas contribute all this and more in the brief time we spend with the women who call upon us.

Lessons learned during pregnancy and delivery can cause dramatic changes in the lives of everyone who is closely involved in the pregnancy and present for birth. These important lessons prepare women for the challenges of parenting an infant.

Women, especially American women, have become isolated and estranged from our sisters. We have lost essential community ties and extended families in which elders were present to pass down traditions, information, and support. We need to be and want to be with other women to share our stories and learn from each other. Only other women can truly comprehend what happens to us during pregnancy and birth. Doulas provide that connection.

A New Women's Movement to Reclaim Age-Old Values

The women's movement of the 1960s worked to place women on an equal footing with men in the workplace. It achieved some of those goals. Now, while valuing those efforts and successes, a new kind of women's movement reminds us of the glory and value of basic differences between the sexes, differences we can cherish as women. We insist on being allowed to give birth in our own way and with the freedom to choose where, how, and with whom the delivery will take place. We had to come far from our roots to learn how inescapable and valuable those roots are.

Midwifery, that venerable trade and skill, is making a comeback. In 2010, the most recent data available, midwives delivered 7.8% of total US births. Removing cesareans, which midwives don't perform, 11.6% of all babies born vaginally were born with midwives. In the decade preceding 2010, the number of vaginal births attended by midwives increased by 20.8%.

Among many reasons is the reclaiming of the experience and process and protocols of delivery from the medical model that first introduced the lithotomy ("stranded-beetle") position. Women had for centuries given birth surrounded by supporting and supportive women. Fairly suddenly, women gave birth in hospitals, where they were often left alone for hours, attended only intermittently by male physicians, many of whom viewed labor and birth as a disease and treated it accordingly: with medications, anesthesia, and perhaps pity rather than empathy and kindness that pour from beloved women friends and family.

Many of our mothers gave up their power in the birth experience by being "put to sleep," allowing themselves to be robbed of their birth experience. As children, we heard those stories and learned to fear birth. An extremely significant change occurred with the regular attendance of fathers in the birthing place. Dad's are now almost always encouraged, even expected, to be present, but many women are perceiving the importance of having another woman present as well.

Promoting the advancement and expansion of doulas is a relatively new idea that isn't new. It represents a deliberate return to the time-honored tradition of women supporting women while retaining the advances of modern medicine where necessary.

Women once treasured their own femininity and recognized their own remarkable powers in their ability to make life and give birth. Those powers and that ability remain the foundation of life and society. Let us respect them, never fear them, and take the time to listen to the ancient song inside us that tells us to accept and revere them.

Finding Yourself as a Doula

In this book you will find information and resources for further reading about caring for mothers, fathers, babies, siblings, and families. A training program begins with the bonding of doula to doula - trusting, caring, and sharing. Knowledge comes second. What we hope will touch you most deeply is the doula spirit, the doula heart.

We encourage you to keep a journal. Look back at your needs when you birthed your first baby, or watched the birth of your sister's baby (or your sister), or had similar experiences. Write down the personal strengths you will bring to being a doula. Record areas in which you would like to improve. Women think too much about their own weaknesses and not nearly enough about their own strengths.

A doula learns to understand herself so that she can help other women understand themselves. As you identify topics in which you would benefit from more knowledge and experience, seek them. Being a doula is a process of continual learning. This book begins a process that will never end. Every mother and family you serve will be your teacher.

Invitation

Come to our party? Join Johnny and *me*?
Time: two o'clock in the morning.
Johnny's the feller who's bouncing with glee.
I'm Johnny's mamma. I'm yawning.
　　　　　　- Maureen Cannon

CHAPTER 1

THE ROLE OF THE DOULA

Societies through the ages have recognized that delivery and the immediate period afterward have lifelong significance to the new mother. Historically, the first six weeks postpartum were reserved for healing and resting from the rigors of childbirth. The mother bonded with her baby naturally as they spent 24 hours a day in each other's company and became intimately acquainted. Frequent nursing ensured the baby's growth and good health. Female relatives and friends made sure the new mother's physical needs were met so that she could concentrate on rest, recovery, and making her first connections with her baby.

Over time, the extended family in most communities began to disappear. Neighbor-to-neighbor support became rare. Ironically, the women's movement had a lot to do with that change as women worked outside the home in greater numbers. Hospital births became routine as the medicalization of birth increased and the availability of women helpers dwindled. Mother and baby were separated by newborn nurseries. Bottle feeding replaced breastfeeding as the cultural norm. The clock, not the baby, set mealtimes. A procession of health care professionals told mothers how to raise their babies. Women often lost touch with the mothers within themselves. Although the traditions of thousands of years melted away, the need for them did not.

The pressing need for *informed* support persists. New mothers today rarely receive enough help and support from their nuclear and extended families. Even when relatives are available, they are unlikely to be prepared to instruct new mothers in breastfeeding techniques or to troubleshoot nursing problems. Well-meant suggestions may be overly critical, out of date, misinformed, conflicting, or counterproductive. One reason is that an entire generation of women did not experience their births and did not breastfeed.

Restoring Age-Old Values

The doula of today restores the tradition of women supporting women during and after delivery. The word *doula*, coined more than 30 years ago from the Greek for "a woman who serves," has come to signify a person who "mothers the mother."

The labor doula is present at the birth itself. (Her role is discussed briefly in chapter 2.) The postpartum doula enters the family home as an empathic, nonjudgmental, nurturing professional who has been carefully trained to support the mother in her chosen mothering style. The doula brings a broad knowledge base that combines her personal experience with the experiences of mothers she has helped and observed in the past and stories she has heard from other doulas. The doula is a postpartum generalist, with understanding of the breadth of postpartum adjustment variables and a tool bag of referrals to offer families more in-depth services as needed. She is well versed in local community resources as well as global research references in order to support a family in informed decision-making. She supplements any assistance offered by the mothers' family and friends.

Doulas help women trust their instincts about giving birth and, from that moment, meeting their babies' needs. Today's doula offers the kinds of information and expertise (but not medical care) that a combination of a grandmother and a caring friend might provide. The philosophy underlying doula care is that a new mother who is properly nurtured and educated gains the self-confidence, energy, and knowledge needed to nurture her baby. The mother is freed to direct her energy to self-care and baby care by the doula's performance of such chores as food shopping, cooking, laundry, and light housekeeping. (For more details, see "A doula's major tasks and responsibilities" at the end of this chapter.) Your major roles involve listening and caring for the new mother without being asked to do so or told what she needs. You will learn to know what she needs and anticipate how to best provide that support.

Boosting Health and Breastfeeding

Many countries with comprehensive home visiting programs have low rates of infant morbidity and mortality. That connection is no coincidence. Postpartum doula care increases the rate, duration, and success of breastfeeding. Doula care facilitates parent-infant bonding, which has been proven to reduce child abuse and neglect. When families receive parenting support from birth, the incidence of child abuse is less than 1%, according to studies by Healthy Families America.

The positive impact of the early support of a knowledgeable doula to assist and guide a new mother in nursing her baby cannot be underestimated. She supports the family in learning feeding cues, understanding normal infant feeding patterns and behaviors, and encourages a father or partner's involvement. By helping to identify practical strategies to aid in nursing, such as how to entertain an older sibling, how to establish a well-supplied nursing area or how to use different breastfeeding positions, the doula bolster's the family's confidence which is at the heart of breastfeeding success.

A postpartum doula's in-home nursing support is also valuable as a referral resource. She can suggest a professional lactation consultant when a mom is struggling, has issues beyond the scope of a doula or simply needs a greater depth of breastfeeding assistance than a doula provides. The presence of a doula can help manage expectations and guide a family to the right care early in their nursing relationship.

Our Enduring Vocation

Looking at the poor state of many American families, with separation and violence so common, we see an enormous task ahead. If we want to make a change, we must start at the beginning: at the birth.

Doulas make it easier for the new mother to care for herself and her family by encouraging the mom make well-care visits for herself and to take her baby to them, too. If a mother chooses, some doulas accompany mother and baby to their first postpartum visits to health care providers. Helping a mom learn how to get out with her new baby and what to pack in a diaper bag for the trip are valuable in giving a mother confidence in performing these tasks.

Doulas teach good nutrition. They help mothers to be physically strong, to recover from birth and to nourish themselves for sensible return to pre-pregnancy weight. One of the first questions a doula can ask when she arrives in a new mother's home is, "Have you eaten?" then prepare and serve a meal or snack as needed. Doulas can also provide suggestions to allow a busy, tired new mom to eat healthy foods easily, for example, putting out a dish of protein-packed nuts, easy peel fruits, and having nutritious snacks and water by her nursing seat reminding her to care for herself as she feeds her baby.

Doulas massage the shoulders of tired new moms and teach them to do infant massage. Scientific studies are proving the tremendous therapeutic value of touch at all stages of life.

When the father or another prominent caregiver is present, the doula gently urges him or her to be part of the family circle. All too often, fathers and significant others are left out in the first weeks. Soon they feel clumsy and inept at changing diapers or holding their babies, tasks at which the mother has quickly become an "expert." Empowering fathers/partners to soothe, hold, bathe, massage, and otherwise interact and engage with their infant(s) is a gift to the family unit. Early teaching and encouragement can make a lifetime of difference to the partner and, by extension, to the baby and mother.

Reassuring Women About Their Innate Mothering Skills

Every mother knows instinctively how to care for her baby. Doulas can help the new mother find her ancient inner voice. Accompanying a mother on a walk, sitting beside her as she gives her baby his first bath or simply nodding and telling her, "You're doing a great job!" build a mother's belief in herself and her mothering abilities.

Women are often highly critical of each other. We tend to believe our way of parenting is the only way. A woman typically hears about "the right way to parent" from her mother, grandmother, mother-in-law, neighbors, work colleagues, and friends, not to mention books, websites, blogs, magazine articles, and pamphlets. Feeling judged and questioned undermines a new mother's confidence and a doula's calm, open-minded nurturing and praise can help neutralize negative input from others.

From a doula, the mother receives the two things she needs most: acceptance and support.

Listening and Communication Skills

While doulas help in a variety of ways, the most important factor is communication. How well we communicate makes all the difference in a new mother's perception of herself.

In general, the doulas role in communicating with the new mother is to be available if and when she chooses to talk about events of labor and birth, breastfeeding, reactions of a sibling, reactions of her partner, or any other subject she wants to get off her chest. Mom sets the tone. You support her, guide her, make practical suggestions drawn from your training and life experiences or from those of women you know or with whom you have worked. Allow the mother to initiate such conversations, and you may offer open-ended questions to welcome discussion when she is ready. For example, you might ask, "Would you like to tell me about your birth?" or "How are you feeling today?" (See chapter 2 under Rest, Relaxation, Support for more questions to ask). Listen intently before giving suggestions, and remember, sometimes suggestions is not what's needed, but rather someone to hear her, validate her emotions and witness her experience.

A doula knows when to listen silently. Listening is a technique to be developed. It needs constant nurturing and in fact is the most important task of the postpartum doula. A new mother is not particularly interested in your birth stories, your children, or how you met your life partner. Listening is an active, attentive process, pay attention to what's going on in your mind as you're listening. Are you hearing her or are you thinking of advice to give, stories of your own or what to make for dinner?

It takes practice, energy and mindfulness to truly be present and listen. As a doula, learn to serve with your ears.

Sometimes a doula's greatest contribution of the day is to hand the mother a cup of tea without being asked or simply to lend a sympathetic ear. In difficult situations, a doula's soothing presence helps relieve the isolation and despair that can contribute to postpartum depression.

Other than breastfeeding, self-care, and infant care instructions, avoid giving parents direct advice, especially medical advice. State legislation makes it clear that doulas may not provide medical care; if they do, they fall under home health regulations and licensing requirements. Providing medical advice that goes awry also opens the door to lawsuits.

Instead, guide the mother to reliable sources of information and other resources so that she can make her own informed decisions. Help her to tune into and trust her own instincts as well. Point out that mothers over the centuries have learned to care for their babies without benefit of books, articles, and the Internet. Give her "permission" to read, listen to others and accept or reject advice as she wishes to suit her family.

For personal matters, it may be appropriate to relate stories from your own experiences or those of clients about the many ups and downs of adjusting to parenting. Storytelling is a fine way to offer suggestions about what has worked for other people and to share the idea that everyone goes through rough times. Marital advice is not in your purview, however referral to area counselors or mother's groups can be helpful resources to share if the mother opens the discussion.

You may, if asked, explain ways to help older children accept the new baby (see chapter 9).

The doula is not a true equivalent of the new mother's sister or best friend. You are in a professional relationship, not a personal one. Don't share too much personal information. Above all, avoid telling stories about sad or difficult experiences or looking for sympathy and understanding, even if you and your client seem to be getting close. You are there for her, not for yourself. Before entering a family's home, take the time to reflect on how you're feeling and what issues you may be carrying that day, center yourself, put them aside and enter being wholly present for your clients.

Do you want to be a doula?

The most important question to ask yourself at the outset is, "Do I want to be a doula?" A fantasy of cooing infants and grateful mothers can be shattered on the first house call when a baby is not well or a mother is angry, weepy, exhausted, or irritable. Being a doula is rewarding, wonderful work. It is also hard work. It is engaging, intimate work that requires a wide range of skills.

Are you comfortable being around other women who are partly naked? The new mother, especially if she is nursing, may be comfortable walking around her own home in a state of undress. Can you tolerate the intimacy required to help someone who is breastfeeding, to assist with bathing and changing a baby, and to bathe and dress older siblings? Consider how you will work with women who do not want you to see them in intimate situations such as breastfeeding or still wearing a nightgown after a sleepless night.

How would you handle being greeted first thing in the morning by a new mother who hired you for breastfeeding support but hands you a pair of rubber gloves and a mop and says the attic room needs to be cleaned? Think about it! (By the way, that kind of intensive cleaning is out of a doula's scope and ideally that is understood before you are hired.)

If you are a baby lover-and most doulas are - could you tolerate not ever touching the baby if the mother insisted on performing all infant care herself? Your primary job is to nurture the mother in whatever way benefits her most. You may be called upon to do the laundry, prepare a simple hot meal, and put the mother to bed with the baby and a cup of tea.

Would you panic if the baby's older sibling had a pet rat? Are you comfortable in unfamiliar neighborhoods? What if the father smoked cigarettes or cigars? Can you remain calm if someone starts to yell, or curse? How easily do you cry?

Being a doula is a monumental responsibility. If you feel ready to be of service to women and their families, you have chosen a superb way to make a difference, one woman at a time.

A Doula Speaks

As a postpartum doula, you will enter the privacy of a family's home. You will quickly learn much more about the family than if you had met them in any other way or setting. One measure of what makes doula work so special is the intimate nature of working with a woman and her family at such a special time. When else could you meet a stranger and within minutes see her breasts exposed as she nursed her newborn? Ask yourself whether, as a doula, you want to be in intimate situations with strangers.

A doula in training once told me that massage therapists often refer to their clients as "intimate strangers." That's a perfect description of the doula-client relationship. We can awaken the potential for a rich and wonderful short-term connection. On the other hand, we may learn things that we are uncomfortable with.

We can and must learn to tolerate and appreciate religious and cultural traditions that are different from our own, but general habits and lifestyle choices may be harder to deal with. Can you overlook a dirty, messy home? What if you smelled marijuana smoke drifting from the bedroom while you were working? If a mother pleads with you to run out and buy her a bottle of vodka, "but don't tell my husband"-and she is nursing-what will you do? These are all real situations that doulas have encountered.

Learn as much as you can during the first prenatal home visit so that you can decide quickly if you and this family are a good match. If not, knowing the other doulas in your community will enable you to make a good referral, preferably before the birth.

Doula care: Fulfilling the Need

The United States health care system has undergone a transition of the venue of care from hospital to home. Currently, what used to be considered "early discharge," a couple of days stay in the hospital, is now considered routine. As this remarkable transformation continues, studies demonstrating profound and far-reaching benefits and savings of early discharge will surely emerge for postpartum care as they are being revealed for other kinds of care.

Doula care is cost effective. It has been scientifically proven to increase the rates of breastfeeding and continued breastfeeding. Other benefits accrue as well.

Doula care:

- Facilitates parent-infant bonding
- Decreases the incidence of postpartum depression
- Encourages appropriate well-baby and mother care
- Reduces the rates of child abuse and neglect
- Increases new parents' confidence in their parenting skills

From the doula's point of view as a businessperson, shorter hospital stays provide a marketing opportunity and a potential increase in market share. Doulas wishing to market their services can emphasize the need they meet for parents who often are distant from family members, beginning as early as coming home from the hospital. (See Chapter 12 for more professional development discussion.)

Women have always instinctively understood the benefits of doula care. Science is finally starting to catch up.

A Doula's Major Tasks and Responsibilities

The doula:

- Meets with the client to establish rapport.
- Makes herself available on the days and hours designated by the client.
- Interacts positively with the client's family while protecting and promoting the mother's and baby's welfare.
- Follows telephone and visiting protocol according to the client's instructions.
- Encourages and assists the nursing mother with breastfeeding suggestions, including alternative positions and methods to promote milk flow and stimulate secretion, within the protocol outlined by the client's health care provider.
- Aids the mother in choosing a nutritious diet. Encourages the plentiful intake of fluids, especially if the mother is nursing.
- Provides information and support to the client and her family for baby care, including bathing, dressing, positioning the baby for sleeping in light of the latest recommendations to prevent sudden infant death syndrome (SIDS), carrying the infant, cord care, and (if appropriate) circumcision care as directed by the patient's health care provider.
- Prepares meals, if requested. Provides lunch, snacks, or both for mother, partner, and children of the client's household.
- Performs light domestic duties as needed to assure a tranquil environment. Tidies up. Does dishes, laundry, and minor daily chores.
- If left in the care of the newborn or other children, asks the client for the mother's destination and emergency telephone numbers.
- Does errands and shopping as directed. For reasons of legal liability, does not transport client or her family, but can accompany client on trips (such as to the doctor) to assist with care of baby or other children as needed.
- Advises the client to direct all questions that require a medical opinion, such as concerning medication, to her health care provider.

Chapter One

Eight weeks *old* and *solemn-wise*
(An *owl sometimes*),
He's just begun to smile-surprise!
His smiles are rhymes.

His smiles are suns that light the day!
The *wonder* is,
The more he gives them all away,
The *more* they're his.

One-two-three, three chins has he.
They're something else.
But when-it's serendipity
He *decorates* the day with glee,
The whole *world* melts.

- Maureen Cannon

Ninth Month

Nothing on earth
Is so very well worth
The g-i-r-t-h!
- Maureen Cannon

The Doula Oath

This oath was originally written for the Resource Mothers Program. No author was named. It was modified for doulas by Chris Morley, who owned a doula service in Valencia, California, and the words have been slightly modified again for publication here. Keep this close to your heart when you finish your training.

May we empower ourselves and the work we do with these words:

I, (state your name),

Solemnly pledge my support and my allegiance
To new mothers and their families.
I will strive diligently to assist women
To experience a positive and successful transition
From womanhood to motherhood
Such that there might be healthy
infants and strong families.

Where there is fear, I shall bring light.
Where there is despair, I shall bring hope.
Where there is ignorance, I shall bring understanding.
Where there is difficulty, I shall be an advocate.
Where there is loneliness, I shall be a friend.
Where there is reluctance, I shall be a companion.
Where there is a need to relay birth stories, I shall listen.

I recognize the confidential nature of my tasks
And promise to uphold high ethical standards
In the performance of my duty.
I shall remain loyal to the philosophy of doula care
And do all in my power to ensure its success.

DONA International Position Paper: The Birth Doula's Contribution to Modern Maternity Care

The birth of each baby has a long lasting impact on the physical and mental health of mother, baby and family. In the twentieth century, we have witnessed vast improvements in the safety of childbirth, and now efforts to improve psychosocial outcomes are receiving greater attention.

The importance of fostering relationships between parents and infants cannot be overemphasized, since these early relationships largely determine the future of each family, and also of society as a whole. The quality of emotional care received by the mother during labor, birth and immediately afterwards is one vital factor that can strengthen or weaken the emotional ties between mother and child. (1, 2) Furthermore, when women receive continuous emotional support and physical comfort throughout childbirth, their obstetric outcomes may improve. (37)

Women have complex needs during childbirth. In addition to the safety of modern obstetrical care, and the love and companionship provided by their partners, women need consistent, continuous reassurance, comfort, encouragement and respect. They need individualized care based on their circumstances and preferences. The role of the birth doula encompasses the nonclinical aspects of care during childbirth.

This paper presents the position of DONA International on the desirability of the presence of a birth doula at childbirth, with references to the medical and social sciences literature. It also explains the role of the doula in relation to the woman's partner, the nurse and medical care providers. This paper does not discuss the postpartum doula, who provides practical help, advice and support to families in the weeks following childbirth. The postpartum doula is the subject of another DONA International Position Paper. (8)

Role of the Doula

In nearly every culture throughout history, women have been surrounded and cared for by other women during childbirth. Artistic representations of birth throughout the world usually include at least two other women surrounding and supporting the birthing woman. One of these women is the midwife, who is responsible for the safe passage of the mother and baby; the other woman or women are behind or beside the mother, holding and comforting her. (9) The modern birth doula is a manifestation of the woman beside the mother.

Birth doulas are trained and experienced in childbirth, although they may or may not have given birth themselves.

Doulas provide continuous physical and emotional support and assistance in gathering information for women and their partners during labor and birth. The doula offers help and advice on comfort measures such as breathing, relaxation, movement and positioning, and comforts the woman with touch, hot or cold packs, beverages, warm baths and showers, and other comforting gestures. She also assists the woman and her partner to become informed about the course of their labor and their options. Perhaps the most crucial role of the doula is providing continuous emotional reassurance and comfort for the entire labor. (4)

Doulas are well-versed in nonmedical skills and do not perform clinical tasks, such as vaginal exams or fetal heart rate or blood pressure monitoring. Doulas do not diagnose medical conditions, offer second opinions or give medical advice. Most importantly, doulas do not make decisions for their clients; they do not project their own values and goals onto the laboring woman. (10, 11) 2

The doula's goal is to help the woman have a safe and satisfying childbirth as the woman defines it. When a doula is present, some women have less need for pain medications, or may postpone them until later in labor; however, many women choose or need pharmacological pain relief. It is not the role of the doula to discourage the mother from her choices. The doula helps her to become informed about various options, including the risks, benefits and accompanying precautions or interventions for safety. Doulas can help maximize the benefits of pain medications while minimizing their undesirable side effects. The comfort and reassurance offered by the doula are beneficial regardless of the use of pain medications.

The Doula and the Partner Work Together

The woman's partner (the baby's father or another loved one) is essential in providing support for the woman. A doula cannot make some of the unique contributions that the partner makes, such as a long-term commitment, intimate knowledge of the woman and love for her and her child. The doula is there in addition to, not instead of, the partner. Ideally, the doula and the partner make the perfect support team for the woman, complementing each other's strengths.

In the 1960s, the earliest days of fathers' involvement in childbirth, the expectation was that they would be intimately involved as advisors, coaches and decision-makers for women. This turned out to be an unrealistic expectation for most men because they had little prior knowledge of birth or medical procedures and little confidence or desire to ask questions of medical staff. In addition, some men felt helpless and distressed over the women's pain and were not able to provide the constant reassurance and nurturing that women needed.

With a doula present, the pressure on the partner is decreased and he or she can participate at his or her own comfort level. Partners often feel relieved when they can rely on a doula for help; they enjoy the experience more. For those partners who want to play an active support role, the doula assists and guides them in effective ways to help their loved ones in labor. Partners other than fathers (lovers, friends, family members) also appreciate the doula's support, reassurance and assistance.

Doulas as Members of the Maternity Care Team

Each person involved in the care of the laboring woman contributes to her emotional wellbeing. However, doctors, nurses and midwives are primarily responsible for the health and wellbeing of the mother and baby. Medical care providers must assess the condition of the mother and fetus, diagnose and treat complications as they arise, and focus on a safe delivery of the baby. These priorities rightly take precedence over the nonmedical psychosocial needs of laboring women. The doula helps ensure that these nonmedical needs are met while enhancing communication and understanding between the woman or couple and the staff. Many doctors, midwives and nurses appreciate the extra attention given to their patients and the greater satisfaction expressed by women who were assisted by a doula. (12, 13, 14)

Terms for labor support providers

The terms describing labor support providers are sometimes confusing. When a person uses any of the terms below to describe herself, she may need to clarify what she means by the term.

Doula - a Greek word meaning a woman who serves. In labor support terminology, doula refers to a specially trained birth companion (not a friend or loved one) who provides labor support. She performs no clinical tasks. Doula also refers to lay women who are trained and experienced in supporting families through postpartum adjustment. They are well-versed in emotional adjustment and physical recovery, 3 newborn development, care, and feeding. They also offer practical assistance with newborn care, household tasks and meal preparation. They promote parent confidence and parent-infant bonding through education, nonjudgmental support, and companionship. To distinguish between the two types of doulas, the terms birth doula and postpartum doula are used. See DONA International's Position Paper, "The Postpartum Doula's Role in Maternity Care." (8)

Labor Support Professional, Labor Support Specialist, Labor Companion - synonyms for birth doula.

Birth Assistant, Midwife's Assistant, Labor Assistant, Monitrice - sometimes these terms are used as synonyms for doula, but usually refer to lay women who are trained in limited clinical skills to assist a midwife (vaginal exams, blood pressure checks, set up for birth, fetal heart rate assessment, etc.) and who also provide some labor support.

Research Findings

In the late 1970s, when Drs. John Kennell and Marshall Klaus investigated ways to enhance maternal—infant bonding they found, almost accidentally, that introducing a doula into the labor room not only improved the bond between mother and infant, but also seemed to decrease the incidence of complications.(3, 4) Since their original studies, published in 1980 and 1986, numerous scientific trials have been conducted in many countries comparing usual care with usual care plus continuous labor support.

In fact, the largest systematic review of continuous labor support, published in 2011, reported the combined findings from 21 randomized controlled trials, including over 15,000 women. (7) The trials compared "usual care" in the hospital with various types of providers of continuous labor support: a member of the hospital staff (i.e., a nurse); a family member or friend; and a doula (not a hospital employee, family member or friend) whose sole responsibility was to provide one-to-one supportive care.

While overall, the supported women had better outcomes than the usual care groups, obstetric outcomes were most improved and intervention rates most dramatically lowered by doulas. According to a summary of the findings of this review (15), the doula-supported women were:

- 28% less likely to have a cesarean section
- 31% less likely to use synthetic oxytocin to speed up labor
- 9% less likely to use any pain medication
- 34% less likely to rate their childbirth experience negatively
- Obstetric outcomes were most improved and intervention rates most dramatically lowered by doulas in settings where:
- the women were not allowed to have loved ones present
- epidural analgesia was not routine (when compared to settings where epidurals are routine)
- intermittent auscultation (listening to fetal heart rate) or intermittent (versus continuous) electronic fetal monitoring was allowed

Services and costs

There are two basic types of doula services: independent doula practices and hospital/agency doula programs. Independent doulas are employed directly by the parents. They meet prenatally one or more times and maintain contact by email or telephone. The doula becomes familiar with the woman's and her partner's preferences, concerns, and individual needs. Once labor begins, the doula arrives when the woman or her partner asks her to come, and stays with them until after the birth. One or more postpartum meetings are included in the doula's service. Most doulas charge a flat fee, and some base their fees on a sliding scale.

Another type of doula service is the community doula program associated with or administered by a hospital or community service agency. The doulas may be volunteers or paid employees of the hospital or agency. These programs vary widely in their design. In some, the hospital or agency contracts with an independent community-based doula group to provide the doulas. Others train and employ their own staff of doulas. Payment of the doula may come from the institution, insurance reimbursement, the client or it may be shared. Some hospital/agency services are set up as on-call doula services. A rotating call schedule ensures that there are doulas available at all times. They meet the client for the first time during labor and quickly establish a relationship.

Other hospital or agency doula programs match a doula with each expectant mother, along with a backup doula. They work together in much the same way that private doulas and clients work together.

Questions to Ask a Doula

In selecting a doula, the following questions should help expectant parents make a good decision. These same questions might also be asked by maternity care professionals who wish to know more:

- What training have you had? (If a doula is certified, you might consider checking with the organization.)
- Tell me about your experience with birth, personally and as a doula.
- What is your philosophy about birth and supporting women and their partners through labor?
- May we meet to discuss our birth plans and the role you will play in supporting me through birth?
- May we call you with questions or concerns before and after the birth?
- When do you try to join women in labor? Do you come to our home or meet us at the hospital?
- Do you meet with us after the birth to review the labor and answer questions?
- Do you work with one or more back up doulas for times when you are not available?
- May we meet them?
- What are your fees and your refund policies?

Third-party reimbursement of doula services

Insurance companies in some countries are increasingly offering coverage for doula services, either as a listed service, through the clients' flexible spending accounts, or as part of their universal health care coverage. Grant funding for doula services is also sometimes available, and, in the USA, some Medicaid—funded health agencies have contracts with doula organizations to support women in poverty and women with special needs. Although some health insurance and flex pay plans pay for doulas, at present, private doula care is usually paid for directly by the client. As of this revision, two states, Oregon and Minnesota have legislation that covers community doulas as part of Medicaid. The U.S. Affordable Care Art, provides coverage for all A and B level research supported services of which doulas are rated A Level in the article *Evidence-based labor and delivery management,* published by www.AJOG.org November 2008.

February of 2014, the American College of Obstetricians and Gynecologists, (ACOG), released a Consensus statement on The Safe Prevention of the Primary Cesarean Delivery that includes the statement "Published data indicate that one of the most effective tools to improve labor and delivery outcomes is the continuous presence of support personnel, such as a doula. A Cochrane meta-analysis of 12 trials and more than 15,000 women demonstrated that the presence of continuous one-on-one support during labor and delivery was associated with improved patient satisfaction and a statistically significant reduction in the rate of cesarean delivery. Given that there are no associated measurable harms, this resource is probably underutilized." With these recent developments, we vision that Medicaid will cover doulas as well as many private payer's as early as 2016 through out the United States. The Time is Now! Doulas Reconnect the Circle of Support.

Training and Certification of Doulas

Doula training focuses on the "art of labor support," that is, the emotional needs of women in labor, and nonmedical physical and emotional comfort measures. The program requires that participants have some prior knowledge, training, and experience relating to childbirth, and consists of an intensive two to four day seminar, including communication skills, understanding of the psycho-emotional experience of childbearing, hands-on mastery of comfort and labor enhancing measures, such as relaxation, breathing, 5 positioning and movements to reduce pain and enhance labor progress, touch, and many others.

To become certified by DONA International, the birth doula meets the following requirements:

- either a background of work and education in the maternity field, or observation of a series of childbirth classes;
- either a background of work and education in the lactation field, or attendance at a professional level breastfeeding course lasting a minimum of three hours;
- agreement to adhere to DONA International's Standards of Practice and Code of Ethics;
- attendance at a doula skills workshop offered by a DONA Approved Birth Doula Trainer;
- completion of extensive background reading from a list of recommended books and published articles;
- submission of an essay that demonstrates understanding of the integral concepts of labor support;
- receipt of positive evaluations from clients, doctors or midwives, and nurses;
- submission of detailed records, observations and essays from a minimum of three births;
- development of a client resource list with a minimum number of entries in specific categories;
- continuing membership in DONA International

Summary and Conclusion

In summary, doulas provide unique positive contributions to the care of women in labor. By attending to women's emotional needs, some obstetric outcomes are improved. Just as importantly, early mother—infant relationships and breastfeeding are enhanced. Women's satisfaction with their birth experiences and even their self-esteem appears to improve when a doula has assisted them through childbirth.

Analysis of the numerous scientific trials of labor support led the prestigious scientific group, The Cochrane Collaboration's Pregnancy and Childbirth Group in Oxford, England to state: "Continuous support during labor has clinically meaningful benefits for women and infants and no known harm." (7)

REFERENCES

1. Klaus MH, Kennell JH, Klaus PH. "Longer-term benefits of doula support." Chapter 6, in *The Doula Book*, 3rd Edition. Da Capo Press, A Division of Perseus Books Group, Boston, Mass. 2012.

2. Hodnett ED. Pain and women's satisfaction with the experience of childbirth: a systematic review. Am J Obstet Gynecol 186 (5Supplement): S160172, 2002

3. Sosa R, Kennell JH, Klaus MH, Robertson S, Urrutia J. "The effect of a supportive companion on perinatal problems, length of labor, and motherinfant interaction," N Engl J Med, 303:597600, 1980.

4. Klaus MH, Kennell JH, Robertson SS, Sosa R. "Effects of social support during parturition on maternal and infant morbidity," Br Med J, 293:585587, 1986.

5. Kennell JH, Klaus MH, McGrath SK, Robertson S, Hinkley C. "Continuous emotional support during labor in a US hospital: a randomized controlled trial," JAMA 265:21972201, 1991.

6. McGrath SK, Kennell JH. A randomized controlled trial of continuous labor support for middleclass couples: effect on cesarean delivery rates. Birth. 2008 Jun;35(2):927

7. Hodnett ED, Gates S, Hofmeyr GJ, Sakala C, Weston J . "Continuous support for women during childbirth." Cochrane Database Syst Rev. 2011 Feb 16; (2):CD003766. 6

8. Kelleher J. Position Paper: The Postpartum Doula's Role in Maternity Care. DONA Internationals, Denver. 2008

9. Ashford JI. George Engelmann and Primitive Birth. Janet Isaacs Ashford, Solana Beach, CA, 1988.

10. DONA International. Standards of Practice. DONA International, Aurora, CO, 2008.

11. DONA International. Code of Ethics. DONA International, Aurora, CO, 2008

12. Ballen LE, Fulcher AJ. "Nurses and doulas: Complementary roles to provide optimal maternity care". JOGNN 35: 304311, 2006

13. Gilliland AL. "After praise and encouragement: Emotional support strategies used by birth doulas in the USA and Canada." Midwifery 27: 525531, 2011.

14. Hodnett E, Lowe N, Hannah M, Willan A, Stevens B, Weston J et al. Effectiveness of nurses as providers of labor support in North American hospitals: a randomized controlled trial. JAMA 288:147481, 2002.

15. Childbirth Connection. "Best Evidence: Labor Support." 2011. Retrieved on 3/17/2012. This paper was written by Penny Simkin and approved by the 2012 DONA International Board of Directors.

For more information about doulas, contact:

DONA International
(888) 788-DONA (3662)
info@DONA.org
http://www.DONA.org

CHAPTER 2

HOME VISITING

Unless you have been hired at the last minute, make a home visit well before your client's anticipated date of delivery. Several weeks beforehand would be ideal. The purpose is to introduce yourself to the prospective mother and allow you to become somewhat familiar with her home before the baby arrives, bringing the kind of chaos that only a newborn can bring.

The prenatal home visit provides an unrushed opportunity for both of you to determine whether you are likely to work well together. The client always has the option of requesting another doula, especially if you are working for a doula service. Personality conflicts should be rare if the doula service has carefully matched doula to client but if you are not the right doula for this family, it would be better to recognize this quickly and to refer her to someone else than to try to be all things to all people and then fail to meet a client's needs at a stressful time for her.

A doula speaks

Learning to recognize when you can't be someone's doula is as important as knowing when you can. By getting to know other doulas in your community, you will be able to help many families by making good referrals and suggesting connections to the support systems that are most appropriate for their needs.

New doulas typically want to help everybody. Yet you are not doing anyone a service if you're out to save the world for your own reasons.

Really explore why you want to be a doula. Can you be totally nonjudgmental? Can you allow and encourage families to trust and follow their instincts? Mothers really do know what is best for their children, assuming the mom is of sound mind and not using drugs or alcohol.

Doulas help women tap into what their hearts tell them to do for their babies. Doctors, mothers, in-laws, friends, magazine articles, internet forums and social media present so many conflicting opinions that its hard for a new mother to know what to do. Encourage your moms to explore the choices open to them. "My way or no way" is not the motto of the doula.

Before the prenatal home visit

You can learn a lot about each client even before your first meeting. As soon as she signs up for your service, mail or email her a detailed questionnaire along with a cover letter and confidentiality form. You may use the samples provided at the end of this chapter, adapt them as you wish, or create your own, modified over time and with experience. If you chose to use the mail, enclosing a self-addressed stamped envelope will make a big difference in whether you get your documents back.

The cover letter outlines the basics of your agreement and asks the client to sign, date, and return it, indicating her willingness to abide by it and to pay the required fees. That way, you will have proof of your verbal agreement. File a copy of the signed page in your permanent records.

The letter will state the initial total number of hours you will work. This may vary according to the client's needs and may increase once her she has a better understanding of what she needs after her baby arrives. The sample letter lists the standard 15 hours. In addition, if you are willing to visit people's homes earlier or later than 9:00 a.m. to 3:00 p.m., adjust your form accordingly.

The questionnaire to be enclosed with the letter asks your client for important details about herself, her pregnancy, and her family and living arrangements. Her answers will give you an idea of what services the family is (and is not) likely to need, such as cooking, laundry, and newborn care. On the phone and in person, clarify and expand on all these points. This may be the last time you'll have your client's full attention after a good night's sleep, so take advantage of it.

Possible answers to the question about special needs during pregnancy include gestational diabetes, pregnancy-induced hypertension (preeclampsia), other, or "none." (See the section on prenatal care and common conditions later in this chapter.) She may be on bed rest for any condition that places her pregnancy at risk. The point is to alert you to any medical problems that your client has been facing during her pregnancy. If she indicates such a problem, consider doing a little research on it. You will not give medical advice, but an informed listener can be more helpful. Empathy and awareness are the key.

From the form you may learn that your client has previously had a miscarriage or abortion. Knowing this in advance can help prevent you from asking inappropriate questions or inadvertently making comments that are painful to her.

One question asks the client to predict her emotional needs after the birth. Some women respond by writing a question mark or "I don't know"; others attach several pages. This open-ended question may bring out very little or a great deal, and is always worth asking.

Once you have read your client's responses, break the ice more personally with a lengthy telephone interview. Set up a mutually convenient time in advance. After your talk, you will look forward to meeting each other in person and will probably feel more comfortable than if you hadn't spoken.

When you set a time for the home visit, say that you would like to meet the members of the family who will be around when you are in the home. Tell your client to expect the visit to last for about 45 minutes to an hour. If your client is illiterate, doesn't speak English well enough to fill out the form, or prefers not to deal with the questionnaire, you can ask her the questions on the phone or at the prenatal home visit, writing down the answers yourself. To protect yourself, however, persist in getting that signed agreement, as with any business arrangement.

A Doula Educator Speaks

When I began working as a doula, I quickly had more work than I could handle. I hired my friends and other women just like us. I felt that all doulas should be clones. (I was very young.)

Then I realized that we were serving women of different races, religions, and cultures. We needed doulas from a wide variety of backgrounds with their attendant skills and experiences.

I learned to my surprise that for many families, I would not have been the best possible doula. It is a relief to know that either the doula or the family can decide in the initial visit that they will not make a good match. I feel much better about saying honestly when I am uncomfortable with a situation and then finding a doula who is better suited to it. She will provide better care if she is comfortable there.

Trying to pretend you are happy with a situation rarely works out well. I often work with doulas on body language. Although our words may say, "I am comfortable with the pet rats you keep in the kitchen," our body language betrays us if our arms are crossed and we have a dubious expression on our faces.

Making the Prenatal Home Visit

When you arrive for the prenatal home visit, learn the "lay of the land." Find out where the family keeps items you'll need, such as cooking utensils, and how to operate the washer and dryer, if available. Once that baby arrives needing attention, moments for such inquiries will become scarce.

It's your job to determine what the mother needs. Quickly and delicately make an intuitive assessment of what has to be done. Ask if she would mind if you took notes in a small notebook or pad. Over time, you will develop a sense of what and how to ask.

Make full use of your time. With your client at your side, and with her permission, open and look through the kitchen and bathroom cabinets. Make a mental note of where things you'll need are stored and take some notes. Ask which dishes your client will want you to use and which are not for everyday use.

Find out how well the family has prepared for the baby's arrival. Do they have enough crib sheets, baby clothes, and other supplies? If not, make a list of some of the things they should buy. (See the section on diapers later in this chapter.) This is potentially a good time to make some practical suggestions. For example, if you notice that all the baby clothes are hung neatly on hangers in the closet far away from the changing table, you could explain the ease of having a supply of onesies and outfit changes when a baby is full of poop and how it would be unsafe to cross the room to get them without bringing the poopy baby!

Be aware, though, that some families, perhaps according to an age-old belief or religious tradition, feel they will "jinx" the birth if they prepare too heavily beforehand. Some won't even buy a crib. If they feel strongly about this, don't press them. You'll be able to manage later and help them set up the nursery and diaper bag as part of your time in their home. If the family cannot afford supplies, learn about agencies in your community that may be willing to donate them.

Ask your client to tell you about herself, her work, and her interests. See if she has any questions about your work or the service you represent. Give her your phone number and to act as a true professional, hand her your business card. Ask her to call you as soon possible after giving birth so that you can clear time for her.

Note: Your voice mail should offer a friendly but brief, businesslike message. Callers should not hear your six-year-old singing a jingle with the dogs doing a chorus in the background. Do not use a religious message; everyone has her own faith.

If you haven't been able to meet others who live with your client, ask her about them during the visit. Learn enough so that you can slide into the household from your first day and take the initiative to do what is needed. Know what the family expects of you and what their priorities are. Do you sense anything that they don't want you to do? If questions about unspoken wishes occur to you, discuss them.

Exploring Diapers

The prenatal home visit is an excellent time to discuss diapers. Talk about what kind of diapers mom plans to use and educate her about the many choices available today. The family will change a large mountain of diapers in the next few years.

A wide variety is available. Disposables vary from the self-proclaimed "environmentally friendly," to super-absorbent, chemical-enhanced types. Some disposables are biodegradable in 500 years, others in much less time. Offer to the parents of the idea of not rolling up the baby's waste in the diaper to be thrown into a landfill but to take a moment to drop the bowel movement in the toilet and flush it away, then fold the plastic and put it in a garbage bag for disposal.

More and more families are choosing to use cloth diapers with or without outside laundering services. Cloth diapering has made a come back and many companies offer varieties of styles, designs and sizes. Familiarize yourself with the different types by attending local or online cloth diapering basics workshops and reading online forums. If the family you're working with will be using cloth diapers, you'll need to know how to use them and offer tips to the family. Find a gentle "recipe" for a bum spray you can share with them as well as laundering tips if they'll be washing their own diapers.

Diaper services exist in most communities. You may want to distribute literature for the services you trust, know who runs any local diaper swaps and add that to your resource list. A local diaper service may agree to act as a referral service for you, handing out your literature on a distracted mom's first week home, especially if you will do the same for them. Some diaper services or shops rent breast pumps and sell baby clothes and even baby food and other supplies for (almost) one-stop shopping for the harried new mom.

As the prospective parents decide which diapers to use, ask them what they would feel most comfortable wearing themselves and you can share that babies who wear cotton diapers rarely have trouble toilet training because the wet cloth makes them highly aware of when they need a change.

With super-absorbent disposables that wick the wetness away from the skin, babies rarely get a feeling of being wet. For toilet training purposes, some disposables are especially made to let children feel wet again, and therefore uncomfortable enough to consider the benefits of getting rid of them.

Doulas should support clients in their choices and encourage them to research the benefits and costs of each option. As with the thousands of other decisions that the parents will have to make, encourage them to gather information, look into the pros and cons of each method, and then make an educated choice. They will feel better about all their decisions if they are made from a place of knowledge. Doulas facilitate the acquisition of that knowledge without imposing their own biases or preferences on the family.

Culture and Family Traditions

To learn to be culturally adept in a family whose customs you may not know (see chapter 6), blend in with the furniture. Don't shake hands or do anything "Western." Ask many questions about religious customs, traditions the family would like respected, how to handle the baby according to the family's belief system, and food prohibitions or preferences for a new mother.

Collect as much information as you can before the birth about practices followed by the family. Monitor your stereotypes; don't assume that every Asian or Asian-American family observes ancient Asian ways. Over time, you may be surprised at what you learn about your own unconscious biases.

Be alert to who believes what, though you will primarily care for the mother. Perhaps only your client's mother or mother-in-law will insist on certain practices. Find out how the new mom feels about that and work through it, but always be sensitive to the wishes of all family members who will be present during your service and remember who will be supporting this family as the baby grows long after you have ended your working relationship with that family.

Prenatal Care and Common Conditions

Be familiar with the terminology of common problems of the perinatal period. The glossary near the end of this manual defines some of these. When a mom says she has gestational diabetes, for example, or has been told late in pregnancy that she has a "postdate" pregnancy (longer than 42 weeks) or the baby may be breech (heading out feet or butt first), your response should be more knowledgeable than "What's that?"

If your client doesn't seem to understand her condition, urge her to contact her provider and talk about it. Doulas facilitate positive communication between women and their providers but never teach or explain medical conditions. The information you provide may dispel old wives' tales and alleviate fear but as a doula, never offer clinical information. If she hesitates to "bother the doctor," remind her that her provider should be someone she feels comfortable asking anything and everything related to pregnancy, birth, her body, and her baby. In addition, the provider will share a very special moment in her life, the birth of her baby, and needs to know about any questions or problems.

Give your client the courage to insist on the kind of birth she will remember with satisfaction. Suggest that she call her provider about any potential problems and to understand them so that she can make informed choices. Women who participate in important decisions about the birth, including the need for a cesarean section, have a more positive birth memory and a lower incidence of postpartum depression (see chapter 5). If your client is concerned about the possibility of a c-section or any other aspect of her upcoming delivery, suggest that she ask her provider for a 20-minute appointment. She should take along her partner or mother to help take notes, ask questions, give her support, and remember what the provider said.

The last weeks before delivery can be exciting and filled with activity as the home is prepared for its new inhabitant (or inhabitants) and family and friends demand frequent reports. Sleep can be difficult as the baby grows and kicks, but rest is extremely important.

Urge your client and her partner to get as much sleep as possible during the last weeks of pregnancy. If your client has trouble sleeping at night, she should allow herself a nap any time she feels tired during the day, as long as it's not so late that she'll have trouble sleeping again that night. The presence of other children in the home will of course make it much harder for the couple to get the sleep they need.

For a client who is still going to work but feels very tired, she might consider starting her maternity leave early so that she will be rested for her delivery. She does not have to return every phone call or respond to every email if she isn't up to it, she shouldn't allow more visitors than she truly wishes to see. Give her permission to pamper herself in preparation for receiving a new life into her home.

Advise your client that for the birth itself, she and her partner will need the strength that can be derived only from rest. Laughingly remind them (as will many of the new-baby cards they'll receive) that it may be a very long time before they get an undisturbed nights sleep again: "Take it while you can get it."

Women and their families often look to their doulas to bring that warm, nurturing touch. Begin this kind of contact with your first telephone encounter and reinforce it at the prenatal visit. Help your client to build trust for her upcoming birth and create the relationship's foundation so she will look forward to seeing you again afterward.

Explaining the Benefits of Labor Support Doula Care

The prenatal visit is a good time to plant positive thoughts for the upcoming birth. Many women fear delivery but may not mention this to you or even admit it to themselves. As they gain confidence in their ability to birth, hearing about the great births your other clients have had may lessen their fear.

Besides offering comfort and support, this is a good time to share information and referrals for labor support doulas. If you don't know any-and you should make an effort to keep lists of all related special services that might be useful to your moms. You can also refer the mom to DONA International to search for doula listings by location (see "Resources of special interest to doulas" toward the end of this manual).

You may want to add labor support to your services by taking additional training.

The woman who has the opportunity to work with a doula during labor and delivery can gain a great deal. A knowledgeable, trained person remains with her without interruption, whereas the medical provider is likely to be in and out of the room, especially if labor is long. The labor doula provides physical, emotional and spiritual support, guiding her and her partner through the stages of labor, and cheers her many small successes as labor proceeds. Penny Simkin has said that the birth doula's role is to protect and nurture the memory of the birth.

Scientific studies worldwide have demonstrated substantial benefits of labor support. The Cochrane Library (2011, Issue 2) includes an update of the Cochrane review on "Continuous support for women during childbirth" With 21 randomized, control trials involving over 15,000 women. [See Appendix for links to the Cochrane meta analysis].

The review found that, in comparison with women who had continuous support, women who labored without continuous support had longer labors and were less likely to have a "spontaneous" birth, meaning without cesarean, vacuum or forceps.

Women without support were more likely to:

- have an epidural or other "regional" analgesia to manage pain
- use any type of pain medication (including narcotics)
- give birth by cesarean section
- give birth with vacuum extraction or forceps
- give birth to a baby with a low Apgar score rating of well being 5 minutes after birth
- be dissatisfied with or negatively rate their childbirth experience (Hodnett and colleagues 2011).

Continuing studies are expected to prove to those who need scientific evidence that labor doulas shorten and ease delivery. Labor doulas also make a tremendous difference to the immediate and long range health of the mother, baby and family.

The Coalition for Improving Maternity Services (CIMS) is an organization comprised of national organizations and individuals with the mutual goal of improving maternity care and promoting evidence-based, family-friendly models of care in the United States. The Mother-Friendly Childbirth Initiative (MFCI) grew in the early 1990's from a collaborative effort of over 26 pregnancy, birth and breastfeeding organizations including including DONA International, La Leche League, Lamaze International, and the American College of Nurse Midwives and well-known individuals. Contributors to this manual who played important roles in CIMS and the development of the Mother-Friendly Childbirth Initiative are Debra Pascali-Bonaro, as well as Marshall KlauS, M.D., Karen N. Salt; and Penny Simkin.

The goal is to look at birth as a natural, non-medical event (even if it requires the use of technology) rather than as an accident waiting to happen. Educate yourself and share with families in supporting this document and organization. Consider giving each of your clients a copy of the initiative as well as Having a Baby? Ten Questions to Ask at the prenatal visit. CIMS encourages the wide distribution of the MFCI document (available free online in many languages). The CIMS website is an important addition to your resource list.

Outside the United States, The International MotherBaby Childbirth Initiative, IMBCI provides the international companion version of the MFCI with Ten steps to optimal MotherBaby Care.

After the Prenatal Home Visit

If you work for a doula service, call the appropriate staff person after the home visit to confirm your placement with the client and to provide feedback on the home visit. How soon after the client gives birth does she want you to start your home visits? How long do you think she wants to use the service? Do you anticipate any trouble spots? As an independent doula, consider and make note of these same questions.

Assuming there are no problems, expect to hear from the client regarding when to begin work. Make clear that she should keep your number with her at all times and contact you as soon as possible after birth, for two reasons. First, you would like to hear a rundown about birth. Second, in order to plan your schedule, you need some idea of when she wants you to start coming to her home. If you work for a doula service, call the office to share your plans after you have heard from the client and drawn a work schedule.

If you are chosen as a woman's doula, she will expect you to be with her and to give her support after baby is born. If there is any chance that you won't be able to keep the commitment because of time constraints or personality differences, make that decision and announce it during the home visit. Once you and the client have made a mutual commitment, follow through as promised for the length of the contract.

Be honest with the women you support. If you can't miss your child's birthday party and it will probably fall during your time with a client, tell mom you will have to skip that day or will be happy to find a substitute. Be open and lay it out up front. To prevent misunderstandings and disappointment, put everything in writing. Women's memories at the end of pregnancy are as solid as pudding. Keeping a time record sheet and asking her to initial it at the end of each visit can be a useful tool, this can include your upcoming schedule which can also be reviewed and confirmed together.

After the birth

Once your client's baby has been born, you will have many tasks to do. Some will be rewarding, others tedious, and still others downright difficult. Other chapters in this manual discuss many aspects of postpartum care for mother and baby in detail.

Know your own strengths and weaknesses, habits and preferences. Are you flexible enough to do things someone else's way? Do you have any problem touching someone else's dirty laundry? Do you tend to feel insecure about cooking for other people? Can you accept the new mother's decisions, such as to bottle feed from the beginning or to stop breastfeeding early, without relaying negative value judgments?

Can you comfortably see women and their families in various stages of undress? Do breasts hanging out of nightgowns bother you? Do you dislike or fear certain types of household pet?

Never forget that you are in her home, helping her with her baby, aiding her in making her own decisions. Consider yourself as a guest who has been invited to help things run smoothly, not to disrupt them.

A perfect example is laundry. A trivial or obvious subject, you say? Not at all. Some people are extremely particular about who sees and touches their clothes and the way their laundry is done. Some moms may insist on doing it themselves while other women are simply thrilled to have it done for them. Some may have systems and notes on which detergent to use for which type of load, while others have no laundry gathering spot and no preferences for how the task is accomplished. As a postpartum doula, you will see the infinite number of ways families live and manage their households. Respect the mom's wishes in all things.

Ask how the family likes to have laundry separated and whether anyone besides the baby has skin that is too sensitive for harsh detergents. For the first month or so, a newborn's laundry should be washed alone, even when it means doing small loads. Use special baby soaps such as Dreft or others formulated for babies. Babies' skin is highly sensitive to the chemicals and perfumes in many adult laundry detergents. Even if the family doesn't want you to touch or even see their dirty laundry, offer to do the baby's. It will accumulate faster than they think. To those who say no, state that the offer will hold throughout your presence in their house in case they change their minds.

Ask families to consider washing all new baby clothes before putting them on the baby. It's possible that the lint from all the new clothes can cause the baby to develop a stuffy nose.

For your own protection against HIV and other infectious organisms that may be lurking, always wear disposable surgical gloves when touching the baby's clothing or bedding, just as you do when you change the baby. The spread of bodily fluids knows no bounds where a newborn is concerned and may not always be obvious. Often, though, you can't miss them! This precaution should prevail whether the clothes are wet or dry.

Integrating the Birth Experience

You are arriving at the home of a woman and, in most cases, her partner soon after they have undergone a life-altering event. During the first 48 hours after birth, the woman is heavily involved in processing her birth experience. This physical, emotional, and spiritual milestone leaves many women feeling both exhausted and exhilarated. The miracle of birth is awe inspiring. Looking at your baby, it is difficult to believe that only hours or days before, this tiny person was inside you and emerged from your body.

Women love to tell their birth stories. In fact, they eagerly tell almost anyone who is willing to sit and listen. Listening is a wonderful way for the doula to bond with the mother. Once you have assessed what needs to be done, ask about her birth story. If she hasn't eaten and laundry needs to be done, toss in a load of wash and prepare a quick meal. As she eats, sit with her and invite her to talk. Listen closely to every detail. To prepare, read Penny Simkin's moving "A Day You'll Never Forget: The Day You Give Birth to Your First Child," reprinted after the end of this chapter.

Even if the birth was not a positive experience, be alert for clues to moms personal strengths. Plant seeds of accomplishment about the abilities she demonstrated. These seeds will grow and bloom into plants and flowers as she takes hold of her maternal role.

Women can never have too much feedback about birth. Even with women who birthed years ago, you can plant a few seeds of empowerment while listening to their birth stories. Women are likely to respond with gratitude that someone is willing to listen and care.

Reporting even a negative experience gives the mother an opportunity to process the birth while allowing you to find some positive trait that she displayed at each step. Acknowledge and validate her feelings, showing empathy, not sympathy. Always listen intently and resist any urge to share about another birth, or your own birth, keep the focus on her and her birth experience.

If the birth involved a loss or other problem, the mother may need professional counseling to help her sustain a birth memory she can live with. Rebounding From Childbirth: Toward Emotional Recovery (see the suggested reading list near the end of this manual) by Lynn Madsen offers comfort and hope from a personal perspective to new mothers who have negative feelings about their births.

Rest, Relaxation, Support

Lack of sleep is the hardest adjustment for new parents to make. The first and most important question to the mother each day is "How did you sleep last night and how are you feeling?" If she is truly exhausted, convince her to take a nap right away while you take over. Adopt "Rest, relaxation, support" as your motto in helping the new mother.

Mothers need to feel that you can handle everything and will take the initiative. Even when they're paying for help, most people feel uncomfortable asking for assistance in any way, even with the laundry or tidying up. Be gently forceful from the start as you demonstrate how useful you will be. Though you are a guest in her home, with a smile, remind her that she need not clean up for you or entertain you, she need not get dressed for you or brush her hair, you are there to help her and not to add more to her plate.

The second question to ask is, "When was the last time you ate, and what did you eat?" Keeping the mother and family well nourished should be a big part of what you do each day. Frazzled, busy new parents may forget to eat or consider it too much trouble but they need their strength, especially if mom is breastfeeding. You'll read more on nourishment later in this chapter.

Here are some more questions that you may want to ask your client during the first postpartum home visit and subsequent ones:

How is your body healing?

How is the baby nursing (or eating)?

Have you been finding time to nap?

Who has come to visit?

What can I do for you? Some mothers will greet you with lists, for others, here are some ideas:
- Breastfeeding assistance
- Laundry
- Cooking
- Tidying
- Help bathe the baby giving mom praise and encouragement
- Run errands such as shopping for food

What are your concerns?

Do you have any questions for me?

Or you may simply say, "What needs to be done today?"

A note for you to consider: There are limitations to doula practice, postpartum doulas are not house-keepers. Know what is reasonable and within the scope of a doula. Feel confident to define that pre-natally and to reiterate it if something arises during your time with the family. For example, if a grandmother asks you to mop the kitchen floor, you may gently and politely respond that that is not something doulas do. If a mother asks you to clean a toilet, perhaps you could say, "That's something that's outside of the doula's scope, but I'd be happy to help you find resources to help you with that." An understanding in advance is helpful to avoid such situations, but if/when they do come up, do not allow yourself to be taken advantage of, it's okay to explain and describe the role of a doula. How you present yourself as a doula reflects on all doulas as the family that you work with shares their experi-ence with others. Some things that may be asked of you may be unexpected but something that is tru-ly supportive and meaningful to the mother. Use your judgement as in the story below.

A Doula Tale: "What do you need me to do today?"

A wealthy mom with a late-in-life baby seemed to be testing me before she would trust me. She would take me into her bedroom and pull cash out of a drawer to give me for errands, as if waiting to see if I would take more when she wasn't looking.

When I came to her house each day, I would ask, "What do you need me to do today?" ex-pecting the usual requests for newborn care or breastfeeding advice or light house cleaning. After three days, mom admitted that what she really wanted was for me to stake her tomato plants.

Out in the yard I went and staked those tomato plants for three hours-the full three hours I was to spend there that day. She was very happy.

There are certain things that people don't want to ask their families to do but will ask a doula to do if they trust you. On other days, what mom needed most was for me to walk around the block with her, the baby, and the dog.

Since then, I have always entered a mom's house asking, "What do you need me to do today?" Never assume that you know what your clients will need. In some cases, you would never guess.

Getting Organized

Rearranging the house around the newborn's needs streamlines baby care and goes a long way toward making the new mother feel cared for. Set up a card table or other small table by her bed. Place nutritious snacks on the table, a glass of juice or a pitcher of water, a clean glass and straw, reading materials, birth announcements and thank-you note paper, a plain pad of paper, and a pen. Keep an eye on the table so that you can wipe it clean and replenish food and supplies as needed.

Set up temporary baby areas in the busiest common areas of the household. Each area should contain a changing table, a piece of furniture that can pitch in for one, or just a changing pad tossed over a sofa or bed. Other supplies to have at hand: clean diapers, moistened wipes, clean baby clothes, a plastic trash can, and plastic or paper bags for the disposal of dirty diapers.

With convenient setups, moms won't have to search for necessities all the time. Those who live in a multiple-story house won't have to run up and down stairs, which they should not do so soon after delivery. For true simplicity, if mom has a diaper bag, you can just keep it filled with supplies and tote it wherever needed. Another idea is to have a basket of supplies for mom beside her nursing or feeding chair. The basket could be filled with a water bottle, handy snacks to remind her to eat, a phone, magazine, and television remote. Things that she won't need to move for once she's settled in to feed.

For a client who can't afford to buy multiples of everything, set up the household to require the fewest steps for mom. That may mean putting all the baby things in the living room temporarily. Assure her that babies don't need a lot of fancy equipment but what there is should be handy.

If the mother frets over a household in disarray, gently inform her that at least for a while, total neatness will be a thing of the past but that you will keep things as tidy as possible. Creating systems and modeling behaviors for the family can help manage expectations.

First baby? If so, you are likely to know better than she does what she will need. Make suggestions instructively but not so forcefully that you make her feel inadequate for not knowing as much as you do. Praise her ideas and validate her as often as possible as she searches to define her parenting style.

Place a rocking chair or other comfortable chair in the bedroom if mom will breastfeed. Show her how to nurse while lying down. (For more on breastfeeding, see chapter 7.) Encourage mom to keep the baby beside her in bed for the first few days to minimize walking around.

Make sure the mother is eating and drinking enough and getting as much rest as possible. Encourage her to wear pajamas all the time for at least the first week to keep her from doing too much. This also gives a strong cue to guests that mom and the family are not in entertaining mode suggesting they should limit their visiting time.

Special touches are always appreciated. Place a small basket of fruit (purchased by the family and taken from the refrigerator) by the nursing chair. If mom brought flowers home from the hospital or some have been sent to the house, ask if she would like some brought into the bedroom. Perhaps she has a flower garden from which you can pick a few posies to cheer the nursing room.

Screening Phone Calls and Visitors

Put a telephone within the mother's reach or remove it, according to her preference. Turn off the bedroom phone ringer and suggest she leave her cell phone elsewhere, at least when she rests or naps and during feedings.

Ask the new mother how she wants to handle telephone calls and visitors. Should you answer the phone whenever you're there? Only when she is nursing? How should you handle unexpected company?

Establish guidelines early, before such situations arise. The mother may be relieved to have you available as a socially acceptable buffer to unwanted guests or phone calls, or she may want you to do nothing at all.

Suggest that the parents record a new message for their voicemail providing the baby's "vital statistics." On the message, include the baby's name, weight, height, and time and date of birth and how mom is doing. The message could state, "This is a special time and we would love to hear your message, but we very busy with the baby and may not be able to return your call for a few days" (or a week or two; whatever the family is comfortable with).

One solution to having a constant flow of people in and out of the house is for the message to specify visiting hours: "We're welcoming visitors between 6 and 8 p.m. on Tuesday and would love to see you then. No need to call first." Some families have also requested that a visitor help out with a single task, or pick up a needed grocery item as "entry fee" when they visit. It would be wise for visiting hours to be at a time when the doula is present to people in, serve tea, and set time limits: "Visiting hours are over. It's time for a feeding and mom has to rest." People will respect the doula's admonitions as a professional and you'll save mom from having to be "heavy" and throw people out!

People love new babies and don't realize how much their visits are tiring out the new mother. In past generations, when mothers had babies, they spent five to 10 days in the hospital. Visiting was managed according to hospital rules. With mothers arriving home from the hospital a few days after the baby is born today, the rules have to be made as they go along.

Nevertheless, always respect the mother's wishes. Some women want to have family and friends over all the time. They may want the doula to help manage the guests and provide coffee, tea, and snacks. If so, fine. Take your cues from the mother.

Be aware of the changing social context in the home. When the mother's friends, relatives, or other visitors are present, it may be best for you to fade into the background and keep an eye on the new-born or a sibling or go do some laundry. Try to protect even the most sociable mother from having too many visitors during the exhausting and stressful first week home. Be aware and help the mom notice, if visitors are delaying her feeds. For a breastfeeding mother, frequency is vital in establishing a solid milk supply. The presence of guests may interfere with a feeding causing mom to miss a very young, sleepy baby's feeding cues. The baby may fall back into a deep sleep and be difficult to arouse.

Suggest that mom slip on a bathrobe for company for the first few weeks. Many women feel the need to dress nicely and put on makeup from their first days at home. That's fine if it makes them feel better, but it has a down side: When people see how good she looks, they tend to sit down and expect to be waited on. Psychologically, what a difference when she greets guests in a robe. People say, "Sit down and let me get you some tea. What can I do to help?" That's more like it!

Doulas can encourage mothers accept help. We grew up with the Superwoman complex. How often if we are sick when someone calls and asks, "Can I do anything?" we quickly respond "No," when really we would really appreciate a bag of groceries, some clean clothes, and a bowl of hot soup.

The same is true after childbirth. This is a time when other cultures through their traditions require mothers to lie in; thus the term "lying-in time" after childbirth. Doulas can encourage moms to make lists of all their needs such as groceries, laundry, meals, cleaning, errands, or watching older children so mom can nap. Knowing these needs is helpful for the doula because when people call and ask what they can do, the doula can list the mother's expressed needs and let them choose one chore. Coming for a visit with the pre-assigned task of completing a load of laundry has two benefits: It accomplishes that load of laundry while setting a time frame for the visit.

People often feel good, even flattered, when they are given a task to do. They really mean it when they ask and are pleasantly surprised when taken up on the offer. If people are coming in and out, you might post the list on the refrigerator (example: "Tuesday night dinner") and ask friends and family who are willing to help to sign up for specific jobs.

If doulas can assist in the rebuilding of family and community support structures, those strengths will be present for the family throughout the parenting years. Doulas model supportive, nurturing, caring behavior. Women who have a doula during labor bond with and touch their babies more in the first hours after birth. Dr. Marshall Klaus has said, 'The doula touches the mother and then the mother touches her baby more." Similarly, our behavior during our time with a mother postpartum can spur her to create models of parenting that differ from what she may have learned as a child.

Transporting Mother and Baby

Never drive the mother or her family, in their car or yours. You may, however, accompany them to doctor's appointments or other places by public transportation or if they do the driving.

As the mother's energy returns, encourage her to get out of the house. Even in the middle of a city, it's amazing how alone a mom can feel if she stays home all day. She needs to be out with other mothers who have babies of similar ages, sharing their ups and downs, and to know that her baby and her experiences are normal. Activities such as a new mother's group or a simple, short walk around the block can refresh and renew a new mother.

Reimbursement for Expenses

Whether you work alone or with a doula service, clients should reimburse you directly for any additional expenses, such as mileage (56.5 cents per mile is the IRS rate in 2013) while doing errands on the job or your small cash outlay on the client's behalf at the supermarket, baby store or dry cleaner.

Make such financial arrangements up front. Reimbursement can get sticky, especially if the mother is distraught about something or you are shy about asking for money. There is no reason for you to pay-out of pocket for the mother's expenses. Prompt payment as you present a receipt from the store is best. Remind her gently. Remember, she is very distracted.

Confidentiality

Nothing your client tells you in confidence should be repeated outside her walls. That goes for anything you observe in her home, overhear in a telephone conversation, or learn by accident while working there.

The postpartum period is a highly charged, emotional, tiring time for the new mother. Revealing any confidence would betray her trust in you. Almost everything you do will reflect on doulas in general. So keep your lips zipped. That goes for e-mail, texting, Facebook and any social media, too!

Appropriate settings for discussing problems and issues that arise in clients' homes are times of sharing with other doulas. When talking about any client, however, do not name her or reveal identifying features.

Safety in the Home

While respecting the family's values, where do you draw boundaries and declare that a certain practice or physical setup is not safe? Some situations are more obvious than others. You'll certainly want to talk with the mother about pets or siblings who are acting out against the baby. Determining where your tolerance stops and your judgment comes in requires a delicate balance. Chapter 3 discusses these issues in more detail.

Meeting the Family's Nutritional Needs

If you are going to prepare food for the family, ask for favorite recipes or meals and prepare them according to the nutritional guidelines presented here. Although you can't force a family to eat healthfully, you can make an effort to prepare nutritious foods. Families eating styles vary, some eat light, or gluten free, or vegetarian or some may predominantly order in. Understanding the extent of meal preparation they expect of you ahead of time and what style of cooking they prefer will help you best meet their needs.

Salads can be bountiful and nutritionally complete. Cut fresh vegetables into attractive shapes. Quarter hard-boiled eggs and sprinkle shredded cheese on top. Cream soups contain more protein than water-based or stock-based soups. The nutritional value of skim milk is just as high as that of whole milk or cream, with much less fat. A handful of cooked grains such as barley, rice, or pasta tossed into a soup with a handful of cooked white beans, garbanzos (chickpeas), or kidney beans provides a full complement of protein.

Be creative. Above all, cook what the family LIKES. Otherwise they won't eat it. You may want to offer to double the recipe for your family's dinner one night and take it to the new mother and her family the next day. Many people find it easier to cook in their own kitchens; if you do, too, ask whether the mom would have any objection. She'll be getting your time for free and will probably be glad-although you never know, so always ask.

When food shopping for yourself, buy what your client needs as well and have it put on a separate receipt for reimbursement by mom. If you are food shopping for your family anyway, you needn't charge your client for your time. If you need to do something special for mom in your home, or food shopping just for her, however, count that time.

If you agree that you will cook for mom's family in your home, ask your client if you may take home the necessary cooking pots or serving dishes the night before. That will save you the effort of taking your own back and forth and risking forgetting them.

Time management is an important doula skill. We often work only three to five hours per day and want to give our clients as much help as possible. Be creative and efficient as you learn to offer your help in the most effective and comfortable way for both of you.

Nutritional needs of the mother are discussed in chapter 4; of the nursing mother, in chapter 7; and of the newborn, in chapter 8.

A Doula Tale: Greasy Chicken

Don't be afraid to admit that you don't know something. Be willing to learn new things from the family or to go home and research them. Here is a cautionary tale about a doula who pretended to know something she did not. Fortunately, the effects were more comical than tragic.

A new doula who was a longtime vegetarian started a job with a family. During the initial visit, they talked about baby care, the baby's room, and breastfeeding, but not cooking. On her first day in the home after the baby was born, the new mother asked the doula to roast a chicken for dinner. The doula had never cooked chicken but felt uncomfortable asking for directions or a cookbook. Plowing ahead, she greased the chicken with Crisco and set it in the oven to bake. Then she finished her day and left.

When dad came home, mom had only glowing reports of their doula. Mom had learned a new breastfeeding position and felt nurtured. Furthermore, a great dinner was waiting. What a wonderful idea to have a doula!

Dad opened the oven to find a chicken swimming in fat. It was so greasy that they couldn't eat it and ordered out for Chinese food. When mom called me, I apologized on behalf of our doula service and offered to pay for their dinner.

Years later, I can laugh at the Greasy Chicken Episode. At the time, though, I was upset and wished the doula had been able to admit that she had never cooked a chicken. The family might have really enjoyed what she could cook very well: a vegetarian meal. Some families love to hear that their doulas have culinary specialties different from their own and are eager to try something new. If not, the mom could have explained what to do or provided a recipe.

It's a good example of the assumptions we all make such as "everyone knows how to roast a chicken" and how wrong we can be. Doulas should beware of making the same kinds of assumptions about clients and their families.

To prevent such a mistake, determine at the prenatal visit whether the family's cooking style differs from your own. If so, mom will have a chance to write down some favorite recipes or to consider which of your specialties she would like to try.

Organizing and Managing Your Time

Three to five hours a day may sound like a long time, but new babies know how to make those hours fly. Upon arriving at your client's home on your first postnatal visit, make a quick assessment of what you have to do. Making a list in a small notebook, pad or on your phone and consulting it often will help you remember not to leave out anything important. As we said before, ask mom at the beginning of each visit, "What needs to be done today?" Then put her requests in a logical order unless she states a priority of her own.

Decide immediately what to do first. If you're going to cook, you may want to get a stew started. If the laundry is piling up, sort the clothes and put in the first load. Note the time to make it easier to remember when to put that load in the dryer and start the next one.

On subsequent days, you may find on arrival that things have changed since you left the day before. Be flexible. If mom is dissolved in tears, take care of her first. The stew and the laundry can wait.

Once you have made a time commitment, you have to show up. Being a doula means time managing your own life. This is a job. You must appear as promised or notify your client if you can't with an explanation of why. You had better have a very good excuse, such as being ill yourself. Be on time, too. Mom may have been waiting anxiously for your arrival since the break of dawn. A lame excuse no-show will cost you your job, a good reference, or both.

Do not stay longer than the agreed-upon time. You are being paid for a certain number of hours. Professional consultants stick to their time limits, and so should you. Doulas often get too involved with their clients, we come to this work because we want to help people, but it is a business and you must act professionally. Managing your time well throughout the visit will help you leave on time. You will improve with experience.

Remember at all times that this is not a social visit. If you take 45 minutes to hear the mother's birth story and you will have only three hours in her home that day, you won't be able to finish your tasks. Combine activities. Mom can talk with you as you cook, do laundry, or tidy up the house. An exception, again, would be if she were very upset, in which case her well-being would take priority over household chores.

Often it is the husband or other partner, off at work, who is paying you to be there. Partners do not want to come home from work after hiring a doula and find themselves shopping and cooking. Provide something visible, such as a stack of clean clothes and a delightful intangible such as the good smell of cooking. Even the family members who are not present during your home visits should feel that you are nurturing them, too.

Closing the Circle: Ending the relationship

Managing your daily time, your weekly time, and the total amount of time you spend with each client is part of being a doula. Another important part of time management is knowing how to end each relationship so that you will have the time and energy for new ones.

In some cases, a doula is eager for the relationship with a certain family to end because they are not people that she would personally want to spend time with but at other times the doula may feel that the woman is someone who would fit into her circle of friends. Make this clear distinction in your mind: If you do occasionally take up a friendship with the mother later, you are assuming a different role with that person.

One of the toughest things for doulas is to separate from the families we like (and the babies we fall in love with). As a new doula, you may find it hard to say goodbye after bonding with a new mom. Many doulas leave on the last day without putting closure to the relationship. They leave the door open so that mother, her partner, and other family members feel that they can continue to call, ask questions and engage the doula's attention indefinitely. Since she already knows the house and baby and has established trust, they may ask her to babysit.

When you start out, you'll have strong feelings about your first clients and may welcome calls from them after your doula-ship is over. The problem is that as you work with more and more families, it will become increasingly difficult to be all things to all clients. Sooner than you think, you will develop a substantial client base. How would you respond if dozens of women called or emailed you once a week? Or texted you regularly?

Many new doulas become burned out by the number of people who have entered their circle and continue to look to them for support and information. Therefore, it's important to be aware of the words you use and how you verbally close this relationship.

One way is to leave a card with a note describing something wonderful that the mom has done with baby or that the household has displayed as a family. In the note, thank the family for the honor of being been permitted to be a part of their life at this special time.

During each day you are in the home, observe and note positive parenting traits. At the end of each day, verbalize at least one, and preferably several, positive things that the mother has done. The first-time mom in particular struggles every day, wondering, "Am I doing a good job? How do I do this?" If a mom truly is a klutz and everything's going wrong, keep it simple, such as: "When I watch you holding your baby, you look like such a contented, happy, peaceful mother."

Use positive words: "Your baby looks so happy in your arms. Look how she is looking at you so lovingly. She knows your voice." That's true. A baby will follow its mother's voice immediately from birth. When you're talking and the mother is talking, the baby will always turn its gaze toward the mom. Emphasize the highlights of what you have observed. You might sense a strong relationship between new parents and how beautiful it was to work with them.

The note symbolizes your farewell. As you give it to the family, say something like this: "I wish you a happy, peaceful life. I would like to give you this little card that I hope you can keep in your baby book or scrapbook to remember me and your first days with your baby."

Often the parents ask to have a picture taken with the doula for the baby book. That's fine, if it's OK with you. You might ask if they would mind sending you a copy.

If this family is ever in crisis, they know your number and can reach you but by saying goodbye and wishing them a good life, the hope is that they will move on to other support systems that are more appropriate after that point.

Before leaving, always ask the family if they are aware of resources in their community (see chapter 12). As a doula, you should advise people about such resources, such as mother centers, Mommy and Me or Daddy and Me classes at the local "Y," La Leche League, and Depression After Delivery (D.A.D.) or similar groups. Some postpartum exercise classes incorporate exercises for the mother in the first half and baby massage during the second half. As the moms massage their infants, they talk about motherhood, parenting, and issues they are grappling with. It helps so much to be around other mothers. We learn from them and share with them on a topic that most people are completely unprepared for: parenthood. Find and recommend local new mothers groups, a new moms meeting helps mothers to normalize her experiences, to learn from others, to glimpse at what is to come and to give her something to look forward to.

Compile a comprehensive list of local and national resources and give a copy to each mother. Keep the list current. Include brochures you have picked up that may be of interest to her. That way, when a problem does arise with breastfeeding, for example, rather than contacting you, she'll call La Leche League. If she's feeling a little depressed, she can call a support group at the local hospital or a D.A.D. group in the community.

Littlest

Sean, Sean, you wear your face two ways,
And only two. In one
You laugh so hard that hiccups craze
Each inch of you. Small son,

The morning's bright with brothers and
They tumble, mini-sized,
Around you, tricks in every hand.
Mid-laugh you look-surprised,

And solemn suddenly, an owl,
And curious. And then,
Delighted by their hoot and howl,
You're hiccuping again!

Two-faced is what you-clearly-are.
You'd melt a heart of ice.
Enchanted with your repertoire,
I love you-twice!

-Maureen Cannon

To a Newborn Son

Solemn-oh, you are solemn as a judge,
Matthew, so newly part of water, earth.
Waking, your eyes are wise, as dark as fudge,
Sober with secrets (stories about the birth,
Memories of the journey'?). But you blink
Hardly at all. Then-quick! -the story done,
Turning away with other thoughts to think,
Owl, you dismiss me roundly.
Smallest one,
There will be other moments, other times.
How we will teach each other always, how
Laughter will light our days, and love, and rhymes,
Miracles all-as you are, Matthew, now.

-Maureen Cannon

A Day You'll Never Forget: The Day You Give Birth to Your First Child

By Penny Simkin, CD(DONA), PT

Penny Simkin is a childbirth educator with the Childbirth Education Association of Seattle. She is the coauthor of Pregnancy, Childbirth, and the Newborn: The Complete Guide *and the author of* The Birth Partner: Everything You Need to Know to Help a Woman Through Childbirth.

This essay became a classic in the field after its first appearance in 1992. It was revised for publication in the 1999 edition of Lamaze Parents Magazine. *We reproduce it here, again revised slightly, with the author's and publisher's permission. The research described here was published in the journal* Birth: Issues in Perinatal Care *(see Suggested Reading list near the end of this manual).*

It happens to every pregnant woman. Other women, even strangers, old and young, approach her in the grocery store, in the elevator, at the bus stop, almost anywhere, and embark on the "When I was pregnant ... " or "Let me tell you about my labor" story. A swelling belly seems to be an invitation for this kind of well-meaning, sometimes helpful but sometimes inconsiderate sharing of "wisdom."

Why do women want to talk about their birth experiences, even years later? It's pretty clear that this day in a woman's life is not just like any other day. It's the day she became a mother, in most cases her partner became a father, and her parents became grandparents. But it's even more than that. It's a landmark in her personal development.

Let's think about the nature of labor and birth. No other event encompasses all these for a woman: pain, emotional stress, unpredictability, and possible physical injury or major surgery. Once completed, she has also undergone a permanent role change that includes responsibility for a dependent, helpless human being. Moreover, all this usually takes place in a single day or less. It's no wonder that women tend to remember birth with deep emotion! And it's most gratifying when women remember these things with joy, satisfaction, and fulfillment.

Several years ago, a group of researchers decided to investigate the long-term memories of women who had taken childbirth education classes and given birth between 1968 and 1974. These special women agreed to explore how well they remembered their birth experiences years later and what impact the births had had on them as individuals.

As was the custom in their birth classes, they wrote and submitted their birth stories to their teacher soon after their first babies were born. Then, between 15 and 20 years later, they were asked to write the story again so that the original and later versions could be compared to see how accurate their memories were after all those years. The women also took part in a lengthy interview to discuss the long-term impact of their childbirths on themselves and their families.

The women remembered very well what happened and how they had felt. The two birth stories were remarkably alike despite an interval of many years. Although details such as the breathing patterns they used and the names of their nurses tended to be forgotten, they remembered other personal "little things" very clearly and described them Similarly in the two stories.

For example, one woman remembered that her bag of waters had broken in the living room and her husband scolded the dog, thinking the dog had wet the rug! Another woman remembered being "mesmerized" by a paper bag taped to her nightstand. She even described the blue flowers on the bag.

She stared at that bag during every contraction and will never forget it. Another remembered the excited ride to the hospital, when she and her husband were singing, "We're off to see the baby, the wonderful baby of ours," to the tune of "We're Off to See the Wizard." All the women remembered details about going into labor, arriving at the hospital, what their partners did or did not do, and some of their thoughts while in labor. They also remembered both positive and negative things that their doctors and nurses had done.

Some remembered soothing back rubs, praise, and kind, encouraging words, but others (the minority, thankfully) remembered being told to "Stop doing that breathing right now," being threatened with, "If you think this is bad, just wait," or having their husbands told to leave. Most remembered the actual delivery and their feelings when they saw and held their babies for the first time. Some remembered large, painful episiotomies that took weeks or months to heal.

Most of the women reported a great sense of satisfaction when they recalled their first birth experiences. Their satisfaction was based on a feeling of accomplishment, of being in control of both their responses to contractions and what was done to them, and of enhanced self-esteem. But more than a third felt quite dissatisfied, recalling that they weren't in control, that they didn't accomplish anything important, and that the birth had lowered their self-esteem or caused them to feel angry.

The most important finding of the study was that the women's satisfaction was not associated with the length of difficulty of their labors or the need for interventions or pain medications. Their satisfaction was associated more with how they were treated by their doctors and nurses, which seemed to have a great impact on their sense of accomplishment and control and their self-esteem.

Nine of the women wept during the interview as they recalled events that had taken place 15 to 20 years before. Some wept from joy: "It was absolutely the best day of my life." "I know I accomplished something." "My Mount Everest!" Others wept from sadness: "Because of what I experienced in the delivery room, I felt powerless." "I was too embarrassed to make a big fuss .... I didn't want to be a nuisance to the nurses." "I kind of blamed myself at one point that I'd had a cesarean .... When I was feeling bad about myself and thinking of all the things I couldn't do, that was one of them. I couldn't even have that baby naturally. No one ever told me I was doing a good job."

It's clear that women don't forget their birth experiences, even years later, and their memories are vivid and accurate, although hazy about what happened when narcotics were in effect. They remember not only facts and events, but also feelings. If they were well treated and given an opportunity to participate, they were likely to remember the experience with joy and satisfaction.

Suggest to your pregnant clients that they ask their mothers, grandmothers, and other women about their birth experiences. Although their initial response may be, "Oh, that was so long ago," urge them not to give up. Questions should be specific: "How did your labor begin?" "Do you remember anything about your nurse, doctor, or midwife?" 'Tell me about the birth." "What was Dad (or the baby's father) doing?" "What was it like when you first saw me (or your baby)?" Unless drugs clouded their memories, they will be able to tell you a great deal about what happened and how they felt.

Pregnant women can learn important lessons from their own research and from this study. Most important is that they will always remember their experiences in giving birth. The memories will be vivid and deeply felt and may influence how they think about themselves and about birth generally. Feeling in control (not necessarily of the labor, but of their response to it and of the decisions being made) and feeling well cared for are more important to long-term satisfaction than whether labor is easy or difficult, normal or complicated, long or short, painful or pain free.

Because it won't be "just another day" for your clients when their babies are born, urge them to do what they can to make childbirth a good memory. Recommend that they choose the doctor or midwife and place for giving birth carefully. Those choices will determine to a great extent how they will remember the birth and perhaps how they will feel about themselves. They should prepare themselves by learning what to expect and what to do so that they will remain active participants in this most meaningful experience. And they should surround themselves with supportive people who will treat them kindly, respectfully, and with dignity.

Twenty years from now, as your client tells a pregnant woman about her birth experience, let's hope it brings tears of joy to her eyes and a renewed sense of wonder and awe at her accomplishment.

Sample questionnaire to send to new clients

To save space and make the questions easier to read, we are listing the following questions without space for responses. In the forms you send out, insert plenty of space after each question.

DIMPLE DOULA SERVICES, INC.

1535 Baby St.
Newborn, IN 46000
Phone: (555) 555-5555
Fax: (555) 555-5556
Email: dimpledoula@baby.com
www.dimpledoula.com

Name: _____
Due date: _____
Address: _____
Contact numbers/Email: _____
Home: _____
Work: _____
Mobile: _____
Email: _____
In which way(s) would you prefer to be contacted? _____

If you have a partner, please list that person's home number if different from yours: _____

Partner's work number: _____

Your age: _____

Are you planning to breast feed your baby? If so, do you expect to need help?

Have you attended a La Leche League meeting or do you plan to attend one before you have the baby? I can give you the names of local leaders if you need them.

Have you had any special needs, medical or otherwise, during your pregnancy? If so, what are they? (Examples: gestational diabetes, preterm labor, frequent urinary tract infections, gained too much weight.)

Are you taking a childbirth education class or do you plan to? What kind of class- Bradley, Lamaze, Cooperative Childbirth Education, other? Instructor's name?

Who is your midwife or physician? Where will you give birth?

Are you working outside the home now? Do you expect to work outside the home after the baby is born? How soon?

Do you anticipate having any particular emotional needs after your baby is born?

Do you have a partner? Will he or she be at home with you for a time after the baby is born? If so, for how long?

Do you have any other supportive family members or friends available to help you after the baby is born?

Does your partner have any special needs that I should know about, such as dietary restrictions for when I prepare simple meals?

If this is not your first baby, how many other children do you have? Please list their names and ages.

If you have other children, did you give birth to them or are they adopted, foster children, stepchildren, or another situation? What are their names and ages? Are any other children living in your household?

What are the names and approximate ages of anyone else who lives with you?

Are any children in your household being treated for any special conditions or do they have any allergies that would be important for us to know about?

Does your family prefer any particular style of cooking?

Does anyone in your family have special dietary needs? For example, if you are sleeping and I make lunch for a child or grandparent, I want to know about any food allergies they may have.

Briefly describe your family's needs concerning the care of your home, laundry, errands, and so on.

Do you have any household pets that you want me to help with, such as walking a dog or changing a cat's litter box? [A doula who is allergic to any animals should say so here.]

Does anyone in your household smoke cigarettes? (I do not smoke.) [If you do smoke, say: I do smoke, but will not do so while at your home or just before I arrive.]

How long do you anticipate needing my services?

How did you hear about my services?

What are the name and telephone number of your pediatrician or other health care provider for the baby?

What other telephone numbers should we have? Examples: older child's school or day care center, grandparents home.

Please list any other names of friends and family including emails, contact numbers, and addresses we can use in case of an emergency. Identify each person (mothers sister, friend in the next town, neighbor across the street). Important!

Please add anything else that you consider important for us to know about you and your family.

Sample prenatal cover letter to send to new clients

DIMPLE DOULA SERVICES, INC.

1535 Baby St.
Newborn, IN 46000
Phone: (555) 555-5555
Fax: (555) 555-5556
Email: dimpledoula@baby.com
www.dimpledoula.com

March 15, 2014

Sally Marner
2828 New England Dr.
Wharton, MN 55556

Dear Sally:

Thank you for asking me to be your doula. Your answers to the enclosed questionnaire will help both of us to focus on your needs now and after you have given birth.

Please mail me the questionnaire at least one month before your due date. Enclose a check or money order for the initial package we have agreed on. Because I must organize my schedule in advance, deposits received closer to your due date may limit the number of hours I can spend with you or may require the flexibility of having more than one doula provide care for you and your family. $XX will cover a one-hour meeting before the birth and 15 hours of home care after the birth.

Once I have received your check, I will call to make an appointment to visit you in your home before your due date. Please plan to spend 45 minutes to an hour with me.

Of your original payment, $XX is nonrefundable. If you change your mind and decide not to use my doula services before the first day of employment, the remainder of your payment will be refunded. No money can be refunded once I have begun home visits after your delivery.

Additional hours may be purchased at a rate of $XX per hour. Hours of service are Monday through Friday, 9 a.m. to 3 p.m. If you want me to run errands, I will submit a weekly invoice for a transportation fee of 55 cents per mile. For legal reasons, I cannot drive you or your family, but I can accompany you to doctor's appointments or other places by public transportation or if you or a family member or friend will drive.

Feel free to call me with any questions. I am often out doing visits, but you can leave a message on my voice mail and I will call you back. I look forward to working with you at this special time.

Please sign below to indicate that you agree with the terms described above. Then return this letter and the attached questionnaire electronically or with my self addressed stamped envelope.

Sincerely,

[Your name}

(Please sign here)

Date

The Mother-Friendly Childbirth Initiative
The Rights of Childbearing Women
DONA International Client Confidentiality Release
DONA International Birth Doula Code of Ethics
DONA International Standards of Practice Birth Doula
DONA International Standards of Practice Postpartum Doula
DONA International Postpartum Doula Code of Ethics

CHAPTER 3

PROVIDING CARE WITH CAUTION: PROTECTING HEALTH AND SAFETY IN THE HOME AND CAR

As a doula, you cannot be all things to all people. The parents you will serve are obligated to learn about safety in the home, how to buy and use infant products, and how to protect themselves and their families against infection. You are not responsible for everything that happens in your clients' homes when you are there or during your time as a doula.

Nevertheless, you would feel very bad if anything happened to threaten the health or safety of a baby or mom you were serving as a doula. Nor would you want to acquire an infection or disease from them or spread it to your own family or friends. By taking certain precautions, you can supply a fair amount of protection to yourself and others, be a good role model for mom and her family, and help educate the new family about some of the issues they will contend with as they welcome a helpless infant into their home.

As you observe each family, you will learn how cautiously they act. If you see any danger, do what you can to discuss solutions in a helpful, not bossy, way. Does the cat seem likely to jump into the baby's bassinet? Even adorable pets can become jealous or skittish and act out of character when a new baby arrives. Is it safe to leave the older children alone in a room with the baby? Help older children learn to start putting away toys that contain small pieces in anticipation of the day when the baby grows large enough to reach for them and put them in his mouth.

Certain precepts apply. Babies should never be left unattended except in a safe, protected environment such as a crib, even "for a second." That's the second when they flip off. Nothing should be left dangling around a baby's neck, such as a bib or a pacifier on a string, especially if no adult is in the room and watching.

All supplies should be gathered and double-checked before baby is put into the bath. If something was forgotten and no one can be called to bring it, the person who is bathing the baby must take the baby along to get it. A baby can drown in even a few centimeters of water. The water temperature should always be tested (using an elbow is the standard method) before the baby is placed in the bath, and recommend the whole house hot water heater temperature is set no higher than 120°F.

Be sure your client has provided all the information you will need if an emergency arises, particularly if she decides to go out and leave you alone with the baby. Review the intake questionnaire that you received before making the prenatal visit. Can you read all the names and telephone numbers easily? If the handwriting is unclear, ask mom for any missing or confusing information long before you may need it.

When the baby is being carried, his head must be fully supported until his neck muscles become strong enough to hold it up. Show mom and dad how to do this.

Mobiles and hanging toys should be hung out of the baby's reach. Tiny newborns look incapable of getting into trouble, but they grow fast. Cords of all kinds - electrical cords, curtain and window blind cords-must be far from the crib. If the crib can't be moved, window cords should be tied so that they are less than six inches long and out of reach. Pins, buttons, and other small objects must be kept away from a baby's reach. Necklaces and ribbons should not be placed around the neck of a baby or a baby toy.

General tips on infant safety are available on the CDC website.

In this chapter, you will read about general health and safety precautions, first aid, techniques that are believed to help prevent sudden infant death syndrome (SIDS), and recommendations for the purchase and use of infant products such as cribs and car seats. By learning the basics and applying them daily, you will underlay the emotional aspects of new-mother care with practical ways to prevent accidents and the spread of illness.

Hand Washing and Drying

Doctors are told "First, do no harm." That adage applies to doulas, too. You will be privileged to enter the homes of newborns and their families. Take great care not to carry any known infection with you or to spread it while there. Protect yourself against infection as well. Your easiest and most useful defense is frequent and thorough hand washing with warm water and soap.

A Doula Speaks

A doula went to the bathroom to wash her hands, but didn't tell mom what she was doing. The doula came back into the room and the baby started to fuss. Mom thought the doula hadn't washed her hands and started to flip out that she was touching the baby.

The moral of this tale is that you must not only take general precautions but also state that you are doing so. The first thing a doula does when she enters the home (after saying hello, putting her bag down, and removing her coat) should be to announce, "I'm going to wash my hands now." Use the sink in the bathroom, not the one in the kitchen, where food is prepared. Ask for your own clean, dry towel or dry your hands with paper towels. Do not use a damp towel that others have used. Rinsed hands that have not been dried can transfer bacteria to food. Dry with a clean towel for 10 seconds, then air dry for 20 seconds before touching the baby.

Wash your hands again, and say so again, before handling the baby each time. "Let me just go wash my hands" sounds really good to a new mom. After a couple of days, mom will get the idea and you won't have to make constant announcements.

To a new mother, frequent hand washing shows your concern not to transmit any bacteria or disease to her and her baby. It's reassuring on the first day to know that you are being conscientious. Make it clear by your actions that this is a part of the way you behave as a professional doula.

Universal Precautions

The medical community uses universal precautions. This set of procedures was designed to protect health care workers and patients from the accidental transmission of disease, including the human immunodeficiency virus (HIV), which causes AIDS, and the hepatitis B virus. Any client may carry these viruses or other diseases. Those at greater risk are women who have used intravenous (IV) street drugs and those who have had a sex partner who is bisexual or has been an IV drug user.

Follow universal precautions for all clients. Do not attempt to decide which clients pose a greater risk than others. You never know-and they may not, either.

One essential element of universal precautions that applies to postpartum doula care is the use of surgical gloves. Breaks in the skin can accept bacterial, viral, and fungal infections; the gloves provide a seal against that transmission. Buy a box of surgical gloves from a reputable supplier and keep a good supply in your doula bag. (If you buy a large box, you can transfer some to a sealed plastic bag. Just don't forget to replace them.) The precise type or brand you use doesn't matter unless you are allergic to latex, in which case, purchase non-latex gloves. If you have a skin condition on your hands or find it difficult to use surgical gloves for any reason, consult a dermatologist or other knowledgeable medical provider about possible alternatives.

You should not be dealing with any of the mother's body fluids in an overt way, but if you change her sheets, you may accidentally come in contact with lochia or leaked breast milk. Therefore, you must glove before performing such tasks, including laundry. Similarly, while part of your role is to encourage mom and her family to do all the newborn care themselves, you may occasionally change a diaper or the baby's bedding. Glove for this as well. Touching a newborn or the baby's laundry frequently involves touching excrement and other body fluids.

Before putting on gloves for the first time at a new client's home, explain to mom what you are doing. She may not understand and may feel insulted at the thought that you anticipate "getting something" from her baby. Assure her that bacteria and other "germs" can go either way and while you will do your best to keep your hands clean, it's impossible to be sure. Say that these are standard procedures used by doulas.

The following discussion is based on guidelines written by Penny Simkin for labor support providers. The guidelines have been adapted for postpartum support providers.

Be aware of the locations of any breaks in your skin: cuts, scratches, scabs, rashes, insect bites or stings, skin conditions, and hangnails. These and your mucous membranes (for example, your mouth and nose) are potential entry points for HIV and HBV as well as other infectious organisms.

Wear washable clothing. Wash your hands and any other exposed areas of your skin with soap and water after handling sheets, towels, or other laundry. Do the same if you help your client change her gown, change her bed linen, remove towels or linen used to wipe up secretions, or remove the trash. Use double plastic bags for garbage and disposable diapers.

If Illness Strikes you or a Family Member

As a doula if you get sick or someone in your family develops a contagious disease, you should call the family you are serving right away. Either let them know that you can't come because of illness or, if you are able, to let them decide whether they still want you to come despite the "bugs" you may be carrying. You may also offer to find another doula in your place. A doula who works for a service should alert her service first to see if a backup is available to offer to the client.

Illness is usually unexpected and is another good reason that independent doulas should try to find other doulas to work with. Life happens. If you can't be there and the woman is counting on you, being part of a network gives you the option to have someone else fill in. If you haven't started your time with the family yet, mom is often more than willing to take another doula. If you have already developed a relationship, she may be less likely to accept a different doula and start over. She may be willing to wait as long as a week to resume care with the doula she knows.

One factor is mom's attitude toward illness. Some clients refuse to have a doula whose child has chickenpox even though she is immune if she has had it herself. Others are open to anything and have to be protected from their own willingness to expose themselves and their babies to contagious diseases.

Don't rely on mom's apprehensions to keep the home safe. Play your own part. Be aware of any disease that you may be carrying, if your child has "stomach flu," you could take the bacteria to your clients' homes without realizing it. To be safe, you may want to ask another doula to fulfill part of the next day's obligation, with mom's permission. Unless you are flat out, you must be the one to call your client and make the arrangements. Never send another doula to a client without obtaining her consent first.

Whoever goes to the home and does the work is the one who gets paid. Work out financial agreements in advance with your backup person. Decide up front who will be paid and how much; waiting until later to work out money issues can lead to resentment. One option is to pay yourself a referral fee and pay the remainder to your replacement. Try to work this out between the doulas without needing to involve the mom, she can continue to pay you as agreed and you compensate your back-up doula after her service.

First Aid

Before going out on any doula calls, you must learn the basics of first aid. You will learn how to deal with bleeding, choking, burn injuries, and much more. First aid requires a course in itself and is beyond the bounds of this book or online course.

Certification as a doula will certainly require proof of having passed a course in first aid. Acceptance into any reputable doula service does the same.

These classes are offered at low cost or free of charge by many organizations. Find classes through your local chapter of the Red Cross, your local "Y," the fire or police department, or the nursing or public relations department of a nearby hospital. If they do not offer such a course they should be able to refer you to one. Additionally, first aid courses are often provided through evening and day-time educational programs ("adult schools" or "community schools") in many public school districts. If you hope to join a certain doula service, the administrator will know where you can take a first aid course.

Your teacher should provide you (at no or low cost) with a small manual of basic first aid techniques. Be familiar with the contents of the book, rereading the table of contents occasionally to refresh your memory so that you can find what you need quickly. Keep the book in your doula bag at all times.

Infant/child CPR

All doulas should take a course in cardiopulmonary resuscitation (CPR), a technique of mouth-to-mouth breathing and chest compressions that is used to try to revive someone who is choking or not breathing or who has no pulse or apparent heartbeat. CPR for infants and children is slightly different from CPR for adults. Learning CPR is a good idea for everyone.

CPR is usually taught in half-day or full-day sessions. To sign up, contact your local American Heart Association Chapter or Red Cross chapter (see First Aid, above) or the American College of Emergency Physicians.

Even after learning CPR, you should have someone call 911 or another emergency number immediately when someone has lost consciousness or stopped breathing. When to call 911 will be included in your CPR class.

Instructions for infant and child CPR and choking, handy to keep for reference, are available at the end of this chapter. Healthy Children is the AAP's website for parents.

Follow this link for a pdf of the Conscious Choking poster at American Red Cross.

SIDS Prevention

Sudden Infant Death Syndrome (SIDS) is a tragedy in which a seemingly healthy baby dies suddenly in its sleep without warning or any apparent reason. The mystery is sometimes solved when it turns out that the cause of death was actually suffocation, intentional or accidental, by an adult or older child. Media reports of these unimaginable situations make it even harder for parents who lose a child to SIDS innocently.

Chapter 10, Unexpected Outcomes, discusses some ways to help such parents cope and lists some helpful resources for health care professionals and families.

According to the National Sudden Infant Death Syndrome Resource Center, since the Back-to-Sleep Campaign in 1994, the U.S. SIDS rate has dramatically declined. Estimates vary, but in the 1990's SIDS deaths were estimated at over 5,000 per year, in 2009, there were 2,226 SIDS deaths. SIDS remains the leading cause of death in the U.S. among infants aged one month to one year. It the third leading cause of overall infant mortality in the United States.

SIDS occurs most often in infants who are two to four months old. Nearly 90% of babies who die of SIDS are less than six months old. Premature and low-birthweight infants and multiples (twins and triplets) have a higher incidence of SIDS than singleton babies who are born at term and have normal birthweight.

Although the Back to Sleep campaign and other guidelines have been developed in an effort to prevent SIDS, these deaths are not predictable. SIDS seems to be associated with a harmful prenatal environment of some kind, but the precise cause or causes remain to be found. The best anyone can do is to note situations that seem to be associated with more cases of SIDS than others, and try to avoid them. Recommendations to prevent SIDS are most important for the first six months of age, when the risk of SIDS is greatest.

Greatest among these recommendations are those related to an infant's sleeping position. The American Academy of Pediatrics began recommending in 1992 that babies be placed on their backs or sides rather than their stomachs to sleep (for naps as well as overnight), stating that this would reduce the chances of their dying of SIDS. In 1996, the AAP revised its guidelines to stipulate back-sleeping only.

The reasons for this continue to be explored. A possible exception: Babies who have certain birth defects or medical problems, such as in the lungs or heart, may be better off sleeping face down, but only if the doctor says so.

Babies should spend some of their waking time on their stomachs (prone) as long as an adult is in the room and watching them. Maintaining a supine position (on the back) is required only for sleeping. Between 1992, when the AAP first made its recommendation, and 1997, SIDS deaths in the U.S. declined by 43%, nearly 2,000 per year. This improvement has been attributed to the widespread change in babies' sleeping positions.

The baby should sleep on a hard surface, without pillows, which might trap air and lead to suffocation (see more under "The dangers of softness in a baby's bed," below).

Studies have found that babies who are exposed to smoking during pregnancy or after birth are more likely to die of SIDS than babies who are not. No one in the household, especially the mother, should smoke when a baby is due or has arrived. A study by the National Center for Health Statistics found that babies who had been exposed to smoke only after birth were twice as likely to die of SIDS as babies whose mothers did not smoke at all. Constant smoke exposure during and after pregnancy tripled a baby's risk of dying of SIDS.

SIDS has been associated with the presence of colds and infections in the household. Research indicates that overheating with too much clothing, overly heavy bedding, or an overheated room may greatly increase the risk of SIDS in babies who have a cold or infection. Signs that a baby is overheated include sweating, damp hair or heat rash, rapid breathing, and restlessness.

Breastfed babies are less likely to die of SIDS than bottle fed babies, according to studies by the National Institute of Child Health and Human Development. Other important risk factors cited by the SIDS Network, Inc., include cold weather, mother's age 20 years or younger, and the baby's sex (boys are at higher risk than girls).

In 2011, the AAP expanded their SIDS prevention guidelines:

- Breastfeeding is recommended and is associated with a reduced risk of SIDS.
- Infants should be immunized. Evidence suggests that immunization reduces the risk of SIDS by 50 percent.
- Bumper pads should not be used in cribs. There is no evidence that bumper pads prevent injuries, and there is a potential risk of suffocation, strangulation or entrapment.
- Always place your baby on his or her back for every sleep time.
- Always use a firm sleep surface. Car seats and other sitting devices are not recommended for routine sleep.
- The baby should sleep in the same room as the parents, but not in the same bed (room-sharing without bed-sharing).
- Keep soft objects or loose bedding out of the crib. This includes pillows, blankets, and bumper pads.
- Wedges and positioners should not be used.
- Pregnant woman should receive regular prenatal care.
- Don't smoke during pregnancy or after birth.
- Offer a pacifier at nap time and bedtime.
- Avoid covering the infant's head or overheating.
- Do not use home monitors or commercial devices marketed to reduce the risk of SIDS.
- Supervised, awake tummy time is recommended daily to facilitate development and minimize the occurrence of positional plagiocephaly (flat heads).

For families wishing to co-sleep with their babies, the University of Notre Dame has put out Safe Co-Sleeping Guidelines, which begins with all of the above recommendations of safe sleep for babies regardless of where they sleep.

The parents of a baby who has died of SIDS are likely to be extremely anxious when a new baby comes along. They may also suffer from guilt when they learn that taking certain precautions might have prevented the death, if only they had known. Such parents would benefit from professional counseling and should be urged to discuss the issue with their medical provider. Doulas should have loss, grief and SIDS support resources available for families.

Preventing Accidents from Objects in the Home

Cribs, strollers, carriages, baby carriers, infant car seats, high chairs, changing tables, playpens, baby play seats, baby gates and other baby "stuff" all cause hundreds or thousands of injuries in the U.S. every year and some deaths as well. The savvy parent researches these products carefully, buys or borrows them carefully, and (not least of all) uses them carefully. No product can substitute proper adult supervision.

The U.S. Consumer Product Safety Commission (CPSC) protects the public from unreasonable of injury or death from more than 15,000 types of consumer products, including many intended for infants and young children. Sometimes a product that has been on the market is found to be faulty or dangerous. The manufacturer may recall it (invite all purchasers to take or mail it back for a refund or replacement) or provide some gizmo that will make it safer.

The CPSCs website is a good source of information about product recalls. Consumers may report product hazards they have identified through a form on the website, their phone number is 800-638-2772.

Consumer Reports, a monthly magazine that does its own research and accepts no advertising, reliably evaluates and rates countless products, including children's furniture, equipment, and toys. Product recalls are listed in every issue. Interested parents may wish to subscribe, look up relevant articles in the public library, or on the CRO website.

Cribs

Inexpensive old cribs are often found in relatives' attics or at garage sales. Restored antique cribs look charming but these "finds" may also be dangerous. According to the CPSC, about 50 U.S. babies each die by suffocation or strangling when they become trapped in cribs with older, unsafe designs or between broken crib parts.

New federal safety standards were introduced beginning June 28, 2011, watch this video on the new standards. All cribs made and sold after June 28, 2011 must meet these new standards, which prohibit drop-side cribs, strengthen mattress supports and crib slats and require better quality hardware.

Crib slats must be spaced no more than 2 3/8 inches apart. Babies can get stuck and even suffocate in spaces larger than that. Decorative cutouts in the front and back panels of a crib can cause the same problem. Corner posts should project no more than 1/16 inch above the headboard or footboard (end panel) of the crib; otherwise, strangulation can result if a string of any kind, such as on the baby's clothes, bedding, or a toy, becomes looped over them.

Older cribs may be painted with lead-based paint. If the parents aren't sure, they should strip down the crib and repaint it. Lead is highly poisonous and flaking paint can be an attractive snack for a teething baby.

The mattress should be firm. It should fit snugly into its space so that the baby can't get trapped in the space. An adult shouldn't be able to slide more than two fingers into the space between the mattress and the sides of the crib. If so, a new mattress or crib should be obtained. The mattress should be covered by a waterproof mattress pad, not by a plastic bag or a large garbage bag. These bags can cause a baby to suffocate if the bag accidentally covers the mouth and nose.

The Dangers of Softness in a Baby's Bed

Is Winnie-the-Pooh a menace? Yes, in an infant's crib. Infants who sleep on soft bedding or surrounded by soft objects look cute but are in danger of being smothered. *Consumer Reports* lists safer sleeping suggestions in this CRO report.

Recommendations on safe bedding practices for infants:

- Place baby on his/her back on a firm, tight-fitting mattress in a crib that meets current safety standards.
- Remove pillows, quilts, comforters, sheepskins, stuffed toys, and other soft products from the crib.
- Consider using a sleeper or wearable sleep sack instead of blankets, with no other covering.
- If using a blanket, put baby with feet at the foot of the crib. Tuck a thin blanket around the crib mattress, reaching only as far as the baby's chest.
- Make sure your baby's head remains uncovered during sleep.
- Don't use sleep positioners.
- Don't use wedges to elevate a baby's head without consulting your pediatrician
- Do not place baby on a waterbed, sofa, soft mattress, pillow, or other soft surface to sleep.
- Don't let your baby sleep in a car seat, infant carrier or similar device. This is especially for younger babies whose heads may flop forward or lean sideways.
- Don't use an electric blanket, heating pad or even a warm water bottle to heat your baby's crib.
- Buy a new crib. A safe crib can be affordable.
- Don't use a crib with any broken, wiggly or missing slats or parts. Don't try to repair a crib yourself or attach strings to the crib.
- When traveling, make sure your baby has a safe place to sleep.
- Educate anyone who will be with baby on safe sleep for naps and overnight.

Infant "Bouncy" Seats

The U.S. Consumer Product Safety Commission (CPSC) recommends that parents keep a close watch and consult the Consumer Reports Bouncy Seat Buying guide. When a child is in an infant carrier seat because the seat can fall or turn over and the child can be injured or killed. CPSC knows of at least five deaths a year involving various types of carriers used to hold infants. In addition, there were over

13,000 estimated injuries in a recent one-year period. (This does not include incidents involving motor vehicles.)

The deaths happened when infants became entangled in restraining straps, when carrier seats toppled over on soft surfaces such as beds, or when unrestrained children fell from the carrier seat to the floor. In almost all of the cases, infants were left unattended in the infant carrier seat. Active infants can move or tip carrier seats by their movements or by pushing off on other objects with their feet.

To prevent injuries and deaths with infant carrier seats, CPSC recommends that parents:

- Choose a carrier with a wide, sturdy base for stability.
- Stay within arm's reach of the baby when the carrier seat is on tables or counters. Infant seats can move when the baby moves or bounces. Never place a carrier seat on soft, plush surfaces that will make it unstable .
- Always use the safety belts .
- Not use infant carriers as a substitute for infant car seats.

Car Seats

Infants should be placed in car seats (child safety seats), always in the back seat, rear facing, from their very first ride. Parents will not be able to leave the hospital with their baby without a carseat installed. Discuss this issue with mom-to-be at your prenatal visit. A lap is not an acceptable substitute for a car seat and is illegal. The baby won't be any safer traveling in its mother's arms in a moving vehicle during the trip home from the hospital than at any other time. Oncoming traffic doesn't know this is a magical ride.

Recommendations for child safety seats have changed a great deal over the years. Many old car seats are considered unsafe. *Consumer Reports* updates recalls and child safety seat recommendations regularly. The American Automobile Association (AAA) website offers information on car seat guidelines. Other resources are the National Highway Safety Traffic Administration's website and The Car Seat Lady.

All car seats must be installed according to product directions. Partial installation, such as using the car's seat belt but neglecting to install a clip to hold a strap in the back of the car seat, is insufficient and dangerous. To prevent a broken neck or other injury in case of a crash, infants under one year old or weighing less than 9 kilograms (about 19.8 pounds) must ride in the back seat, facing the rear of the vehicle. A child safety seat must never be installed in the front seat of a vehicle equipped with air bags. The force of an inflating air bag can kill an infant. Warn your clients that infant carrier seats are not to be used in a car unless the directions specifically state that the seat may be used for both purposes. Simply buckling the seat into a seat belt is not enough.

All passenger vehicles model year 2003 and newer now have to be equipped with top and lower anchors to which child safety seats can be attached in a simple and uniform way. LATCH stands for Lower Anchors and Tethers for Children. In Canada it is known as LUAS (Lower Universal Anchorage System). The LATCH system secures a carseat to the vehicle using straps from the child safety seat that connect to metal anchors in the car/truck. Vehicles model year 2003 and newer must have lower anchors in at least two positions and tether anchors in at least three positions.

All 50 states and the District of Columbia have passed mandatory (but inconsistent) child safety seat usage laws for young children. Failing to follow them can incur a ticket as well as danger to the child. Many local fire or police departments run car seat installations clinics in which certified professionals install car seats for families. Look into these in your area and provide recommendations to your clients.

CPR for Infants (Age < 1)

If you are alone with the infant give 2 minutes of CPR before calling 911.

1. Shout and Tap: Shout and gently tap the child on the shoulder. If there is no response and not breathing or not breathing normally, position the infant on his or her back and begin CPR.

2. Give 30 Compressions: Give 30 gentle chest compressions at the rate of at least 100 per minute. Use two or three fingers in the center of the chest just below the nipples. Press down approximately one-third the depth of the chest (about 1 and a half inches).

3. Open The Airway: Open the airway using a head tilt lifting of chin. Do not tilt the head too far back

4. Give 2 Gentle Breaths: If the baby is not breathing or not breathing normally, cover the baby's mouth and nose with your mouth and give 2 gentle breaths. Each breath should be 1 second long. You should see the baby's chest rise with each breath.

CONTINUE WITH 30 PUMPS AND 2 BREATHS UNTIL HELP ARRIVES

For full instructions with graphics please visit University of Washington School of Medicine Infant CPR.

CHAPTER 4

HONORING POSTPARTUM WOMEN AND TEACHING SELF-CARE

Women are often surprised and disappointed by the way their bodies look and feel after childbirth. The baby's out-why hasn't everything returned to normal? Reassure mom that these changes *are* normal and that you will help her start to regain a body image that is acceptable to her. Many such body changes will be discussed in this chapter.

Stitches, bleeding, breast care ... why are we telling you all this? To remind you that your role is to provide information and to give you important background.

Mothers must do all self-care on their own bodies. Doulas should not touch sanitary pads, discharge, sutures, or cesarean section scars, but there are moments when mothers feel they need to share some of their private pains and aches with another woman. They often ask, "Does this look normal?" Be prepared to distinguish between normal and abnormal.

You might say, "From my own experience and from working with other mothers, I have seen that this soreness happens all the time. It's often normal but if you're concerned, double check with your provider because I'm not a medical provider."

Assure mom that if she has a question or concern at any time, she should contact her provider. She is entitled to that professional's advice. From your own perspective, a doula who pronounced something fine that *wasn't* fine would open herself and her service to lawsuits, not to mention the possibility of allowing a problem to worsen without appropriate medical attention.

A nervous new mom may fret about "bothering the doctor or midwife." Remind her that that is what the provider is there for and that health care providers expect occasional phone calls from their patients. The provider may not always be able to come to the phone, but the nurses and other personnel who answer mom's call are well trained, can answer most questions, and know when to consult the provider.

If mom is not satisfied with the answer, she can insist on speaking directly with the provider. She should realize that unless the situation is an emergency, the provider may not call back for a while, possibly after the day's office visits have ended. Many pediatricians have "calling hours," typically in the early morning, when they make themselves available for patients' questions.

Mom should call her provider immediately if she experiences any of these danger signs:

- Pain in her legs when she stands or walks
- Fever higher than 100° F, with or without chills
- Very heavy bleeding (twice the amount of the heaviest day of her normal menstrual period)
- The passing of large clots
- Foul-smelling vaginal discharge
- Abdominal tenderness
- Continued difficulty urinating or pain or burning while urinating
- Swelling, redness, or tenderness in one area of the breast
- After a cesarean section or episiotomy, look for all the above, plus:
- Oozing or redness at the incision site
- Foul-smelling discharge at the incision site
- Any gaping or opening of the incision

The Uterus and Afterpains

Immediately after delivery, the top of the uterus is roughly on a level with the navel. It shrinks slightly every day. By the end of the first week, it should be almost down to the hairline. Mom should check the uterus daily. It should stay firm, get smaller every day, and not hurt when touched from the outside. Any symptom of a uterine infection should be reported to the medical provider: the uterus feels soft instead of hard, the top doesn't move down every day, the uterus feels tender when touched, or mom develops abdominal pain or a fever. Excessive cramping, especially if accompanied by heavier-than-average bleeding, may be a sign of retained membranes or fragments of the placenta. (If a mother's milk is taking longer than the usual 3-4 days to "come in," this could be another sign of retained placenta.)

Cramping of the uterus (afterpains) is normal for two to three days after delivery. These cramps may be stronger with each pregnancy as the previously stretched uterus works harder to return to its normal shape and size. Breastfeeding can increase cramping by triggering the release of oxytocin, a hormone that stimulates uterine contractions. Congratulate the breastfeeding mom on helping her uterus to return to its normal size. Cramping also helps to minimize bleeding. It can be difficult for hurting moms to think of something good about feeling bad. Your attitude and pep talks can help a lot.

If cramping becomes uncomfortable, advise mom to urinate more often. A full bladder increases uterine contractions. Slow, deep breathing and relaxation techniques used for labor contractions can help relieve pain and help moms manage afterpains. Lying on the stomach with a small pillow placed directly under the uterus may bring relief. The cramps tend to get much worse for about 10 minutes and then disappear.

By the second day after delivery, warm blankets may be applied to mom's abdomen. These are comforting and may relieve cramping. If pain persists, mom can ask her medical provider for permission to take pain medication such as Tylenol or ibuprofen.

Vaginal Discharge and Bleeding

The placenta that was attached to the inside of the uterus emerges through the vagina after delivery and is then, along with the emerging membranes, called the afterbirth. After the placenta has emerged, a bright red fluid called lochia begins to flow. Tell mom that this discharge is normal and indicates healing and regeneration of the uterine lining. Any time you can put a positive spin on something that starts out being distressing, you have made an important contribution to a new mother's sense of comfort in the first week.

A gush of dark red blood after the mother has been lying down is a normal result of vaginal pooling. She should be prepared for this so that she doesn't stain her clothes, bedclothes, furniture, or carpeting and especially so that she won't be frightened.

Women should not douche or use tampons during the postpartum period. Many women have not explored sanitary pad options for years and may not realize how many kinds are available. The large, super-absorbent kind with "wings" are great. Give mom permission to use as many as she needs and to change pads whenever she wants, and at least every two to three hours. Used pads should be placed in a sanitary receptacle such as a plastic bag (keep one in the bedroom and one in the bathroom) or a wastebasket lined with a plastic garbage bag. Washing her hands after each change is a good idea.

About seven or eight days after delivery, the lochia should look more pink than red. It may look pink or brown for another week to 10 days and finally become slight brownish spotting. After two or three weeks the lochia becomes creamy yellow.

The volume decreases gradually and about three to six weeks after delivery, lochia stops. Reasons to call the provider include soaking a pad more often than every two hours on the first day after birth or every four hours on any subsequent day.

Some spotting for up to six weeks postpartum is normal. Bleeding that suddenly becomes heavy and bright red or that resumes after it has begun to fade away is a sign that the new mother may be over-exerting herself. Encourage her to lie down and put her feet up for at least one to two hours and preferably longer. If heavy bleeding continues, she should call her medical provider. Another reason to call the provider at any time is if the lochia smells bad, not merely like blood or a normal menstrual period. A foul smell may signify an infection.

When women insist on doing a great deal at home for the first weeks after delivery, lochia may continue to flow for a longer time. To prevent such problems is only one of many reasons that new mothers should rest all they can and never overexert themselves. The help of family, friends, and doulas is important in a mother's physical recovery from birth.

Stitches from a Tear or an Episiotomy

Applying ice or cold packs to the site of a repair of a tear or an episiotomy for the first 12 to 24 hours after delivery can prevent or relieve pain, swelling, and bleeding. After that, moderate heat works best. Simply repositioning the sanitary pad so that it doesn't rub against the stitches may help, too. Suggest that mom lie on her side instead of sitting some of the time.

Here's an excellent tip for the sore new mom: Buy a bottle of witch hazel at any drugstore. Pour just a little on a sanitary napkin—enough to make the pad slightly damp, but not drenched. It still has to be absorbent. Place the pad in a plastic bag. Repeat, using the same bag, with two or three additional pads. Place the bag and the bottle of witch hazel in the refrigerator.

When it's time for mom to change her sanitary pad, she uses one of these. The coolness feels great against a perineum (area around the vagina and extending to the anus) that's tender and sore, with or without a tear or an episiotomy, and helps to reduce swelling; the witch hazel promotes healing. Tell mom that this method works for hemorrhoids, too.

Mom will have to change pads more often with this method, but she'll want to anyway because the coolness lasts for only about 20 minutes. More frequent changes are a fine idea, since they remove bacteria from the area, reducing the chances of infection. If the stitches are very sore, suggest a sitz bath (soaking in a small tub of warm-not hot-water) or a soak in a warm bath two or three times a day if the medical provider permits. Soaking softens the stitches and promotes circulation, decreasing discomfort. Each soak should last for no more than about 15 to 20 minutes. To prevent infection, make sure the tub or sitz bath is very clean.

A natural remedy for perineal soreness is to soak a tea bag of comfrey root in hot water until it has expanded and absorbed most of the water. Place the teabag, which has become slightly gooey, on the perineum three times a day for approximately 20 minutes. Alternatively, add the teabag to the sitz bath. A hand-held hair dryer on "low" is good for drying the perineum after bathing. The stitches will dissolve by themselves. Mild heat, air, and Kegel exercises all promote healing.

Squeezing the buttocks together before sitting down minimizes perineal discomfort. Mom may want to sit on a pillow protected against the possible leakage of vaginal discharge and bleeding (see below) by a small plastic-coated bed pad like the ones used in hospitals or any sheet of plastic.

Episiotomy stitches dissolve one to three weeks after delivery. Alert mom that as this happens, she may find bits of thread on her sanitary pads or toilet paper.

After a Cesarean Section

A mother who has undergone a cesarean delivery has special needs. She shouldn't wear anything snug over the incision for a few weeks. She should hold a pillow over the incision when feeding the baby. She should not lift anything heavier than the baby for at least two to three weeks.

The woman who has had a c-section can walk and move around as tolerated but should not overdo it. She will have lochia for about the first 10 days (or longer, if she is breastfeeding). She should rest, rest, rest; drink plenty of fluids-maybe more than she really wants; eat to taste; and take a good multivitamin (approved by her provider) daily.

As a doula, be extra-sensitive to the fact that this mom has experienced both major surgery and birth at the same time. Many women who have had c-sections become very frustrated at weeks 2 to 3 when they talk to friends who are up and out and they're still struggling. From the doula perspective, give her extra TLC. Many mothers with c-sections are hard on themselves because they don't fully realize they have given birth and had major surgery. Remind mom that she has a double whammy to recover from and it will take longer than if she had delivered vaginally. Praise her for giving an extra measure of her own comfort to her baby's well-being.

Some women who have had c-sections say they feel like failures because they didn't give birth naturally, especially if they had planned on an unmediated childbirth and dreamed all kinds of romantic things about the birth. These moms are no less "real women" or "real moms" than those whose babies emerged through the vaginal canal. Somehow that can be obvious to everyone but them.

What really influences their feelings, however, is more likely to depend on how they were treated and whether they were part of the decision making. If they didn't feel respected or if they believe that things were done to them, rather than by them, the experience can be negative even if the birth went fine and the baby is healthy. You may be surprised to hear real anger from healthy women with healthy babies mostly related to what people, especially health care professionals, said or didn't say. All this can be true for the woman who delivered vaginally, too.

As a doula, listen to these women. Don't dismiss or negate any of their feelings. Being allowed to process the birth, whether positively or negatively, is extremely important. While empathizing, listen for the positive things that they did do to influence the birthing process. For more on this, see "Integrating the birth experience" in chapter 2. Many women need to be given "permission" to both feel grateful for a healthy baby while also grieving the loss of the birth experience she envisioned.

On a practical note, a woman who has had a c-section typically suffers from gas pains for a while. To relieve these pains, she can lie on her left side with her knees bent and slowly knead her abdomen. When standing, she should stand tall, tightening her abdominal muscles and breathing deeply, to help the gas bubbles move through her system.

After a Tubal Ligation

If your client has taken the opportunity of being in the hospital to undergo surgical sterilization (a tubal ligation, or "having her [fallopian] tubes tied"), and everything else is normal, she can safely resume most activities, including bathing, driving, and light household tasks, within a few days. No activity should be strenuous enough to cause pain, however, and rest to prevent fatigue is the watchword. She should not resume an exercise program of any kind without her providers permission.

If sutures are rubbing irritatingly against the patient's underwear, she can apply a small plastic adhesive bandage such as a Band-Aid to protect the area.

It's okay for her to wash the incision gently with a little soap and water during a shower or bath, then rinse and pat dry afterward. The rest of the time, the incision should be kept dry. If the area over her bellybutton (navel) or around the incision is a little tender or even a little red, it's probably okay but real soreness or extensive redness may indicate an infection as can chills or fever over 99.6°F. Mom should observe the site carefully and report to her medical provider any drainage or symptoms that worry her.

Bathing and Shampooing

Women tend to perspire more than usual after delivery and are eager to cleanse themselves. Some physicians do not allow women to take tub baths until after their postpartum checkups (especially if an episiotomy has been performed) but do permit sitz baths and showers sooner after delivery. Midwives do tend to encourage tub baths. Always follow the instructions of your client's provider, not your own preferences and opinions.

Heat can accelerate blood flow. Therefore, hot, steamy baths and showers should be avoided soon after delivery. Mom should ask her provider when she may take a hot bath again. Heat also promotes the flow of breast milk, so bottle feeding moms in particular should avoid hot baths until milk is no longer flowing. Breastfeeding moms, too, should limit their breasts' exposure to hot water (see "Basic breast care" later in this chapter). Hair washing is not a problem if done in a sink. New moms may wash their hair whenever they wish.

Urinating and Wiping

Many women, especially those with tender perineums, feel very nervous about urinating for the first couple of days after birth. They may fear that the urine will burn the delicate skin or may just be uncomfortable with the way they feel in general. In any case, they may confide such feelings only to their doulas. They may not mention this even to their medical providers or partners. As doulas we can offer some practical comfort measures.

To help a mom urinate while sitting on the toilet, suggest running the water in the bathroom sink or shower or use a few drops of peppermint oil on a cloth or dropped into the toilet water. If that doesn't work, or if she needs to bathe anyway, suggest that she may feel more comfortable standing under a warm shower when she feels the need to urinate, which she should do often. This sounds simple but women rarely think of it themselves. It works! The warm water washes them off immediately and cleans the shower.

When leaving the hospital, mom may have been given a plastic bottle with a nozzle. (These can also be purchased inexpensively.) Mom fills the bottle with warm water on her way to the toilet. After urinating or having a bowel movement, she squirts the warm water over the perineal area instead of using toilet paper, which may be too abrasive in the early days after birth. She then gently pats herself dry (sutures in particular should not be left damp, a condition that might foster bacterial growth and infection) or can use a blow dryer on low heat.

Another wiping method is to keep a roll of soft, high-quality paper towels in the bathroom and fold a sheet into a flat square for each use. She moistens a sheet with warm water as needed and uses it to pat the perineal area clean. As always, she should pat or wipe from front to back.

Bowel Movements and Constipation

Moms often worry that their episiotomy stitches or hemorrhoids will tear open or that they will feel pain if they have a bowel movement, and consciously or subconsciously suppress the urge to "go." Remind mom that she'll do best if she answers nature's call promptly. Some women really don't need to have a bowel movement for three to five days after birth and shouldn't worry about it.

For many women, bowel movements are difficult to pass for the first weeks after delivery. Mention this to your client, who may not feel comfortable bringing it up. If she is constipated, she will be glad to hear that the problem is normal and can resolve soon.

Suggest that she eat plenty of high-fiber foods, such as bran and whole-grain cereals and breads. Raw fruits and vegetables promote the digestive process and are low fat and low calorie. Prepare these foods for her and explain why they will help.

Drinking plenty of water is important for new moms at all times, but additionally to relieve constipation. An intake of ample fluids is crucial for the breastfeeding mother as well. Even walking around keeps the digestive system working. As mom, holding her baby against her shoulder, walks around and around the room to put the baby to sleep, she is helping her digestive tract to work properly, too.

A mom with constipation should take her time in the bathroom. Tell her that you will watch the baby and she should sit there as long as she needs to. Reading a book or magazine may help her muscles relax. Children's books are good for this! Advise mom to avoid straining while having a bowel movement.

Nursing mothers should not take strong laxatives, which can cause the baby to have diarrhea. If foods and liquids don't relieve mom's constipation and she is very distressed, suggest that she call her provider. The provider may prescribe a stool softener mild laxative such as milk of magnesium may be acceptable, even for a nursing mother, but only with the provider's permission. Tell her to be sure to mention that she is nursing the baby.

Hemorrhoids

Varicose veins near the rectum, called hemorrhoids, can become more prominent after a vaginal birth when the woman has had to "bear down," placing stress on the area. Hemorrhoids that appear for the first time late in pregnancy or after delivery tend to heal on their own. Until then, suggest these methods to reduce discomfort:

- Take frequent sitz baths for up to 20 minutes at a time.
- Avoid straining during bowel movements.
- Drink plenty of fluids (six to eight large glasses a day).
- Eat raisins, figs, dates, prunes or prune juice, citrus fruits and juices, whole grains, green vegetables, and other time-honored natural stool softeners and high-fiber foods.
- If the pain persists, mom can ask her provider for pain medication or an anesthetic cream or ointment to apply to the painful area gently.
- Take one 50-milligram capsule of vitamin B6 daily.
- Apply comfrey root compresses or wear sanitary napkins with a little witch hazel applied, then refrigerated (see under "Stitches from an episiotomy," above).

For sore hemorrhoids, mom may ask her medical provider to recommend or prescribe an ointment.

One birthing center suggests that moms mix two ointments, hydrocortisone and 5% Xylocaine, in the palm of the hand and apply the mixture to hemorrhoids externally.

Basic Breast Care

All newly delivered women should expect some degree of fullness on the second to fourth day after birth. The breasts become full and may feel heavy, hard, and painful. This extreme fullness usually lasts for 48 to 72 hours.

Many women who are not breastfeeding find they can minimize their discomfort by wearing a snug, well-fitting brassiere (such as a cotton sports bra or a maternity bra) day and night for a week or two, until the milk supply has receded. If the bra only makes her feel worse, forget it. Placing cold compresses or ice packs on the breasts for an hour three or four times a day relieves aching. Assure mom that the most uncomfortable period lasts for only about 36 hours. Bottle feeding mothers should not attempt to relieve the pressure by pumping or expressing milk. This would only tell the body to make more. Mom can also ask an herbalist or lactation consultant for help in decreasing milk supply.

Nursing moms can prevent or relieve early engorgement by nursing every hour and a half to two hours. Emptying the breast decreases the feeling of fullness while stimulating milk production. Moderate heat to the rescue: Warm compresses, standing in a warm (not hot) shower, and using a hair dryer on the low setting feel good. Preventing engorgement is important as engorgement can inhibit milk supply.

After the first few days, breastfeeding may involve some tenderness but should not hurt severely or continuously. When a nursing mom feels real pain, however, something is wrong. She should contact her health care provider or lactation consultant. The most common cause is poor latch-on, which can be corrected quite easily (again, please see chapter 7). Proper positioning and breaking the suction before removing the baby from the breast protect the nipples against cracking and bleeding.

The bottle feeding mom should take care not to stimulate her breasts, which would trigger the discharge of milk. In the shower, she should turn her back to the flow of water so that warm water doesn't flow onto her breasts. During love play, her partner should touch her breasts very gently, if at all, until milk production has stopped.

Continuous support from a sturdy bra is recommended for nursing mothers. The breasts are larger and heavier when filled with milk. Nursing bras have cups like flaps that unclip and open for baby so that they don't have to be removed for breastfeeding. Nursing pads can be inserted in the cups between feedings to absorb any milk leakage. If mom prefers to wear no bra at all and feels comfortable that way, fine. An overly tight bra would feel worse than none at all and can cause plugged ducts.

With their medical provider's permission, both breastfeeding and bottle feeding mothers may take Tylenol as needed for discomfort. A folk remedy that many women swear by consists of wrapping engorged breasts in clean, raw cabbage leaves. Lactation consultants have said that this method brings rapid relief of discomfort and even facilitates the flow of breast milk.

The nursing mother should bathe her breasts with plain water only. Soap, alcohol, and lotion are overly drying to the skin and nipples, making any pain or damage worse. Strong soaps remove protective oils in the skin. She may wash the rest of her body with soap as usual, however.

There is no need to apply creams or oils to the breasts or nipples. If mom feels discomfort and asks what she can do, suggest that she rub a little expressed breast milk into the nipples gently after each feeding and let them air dry. (This is a good preventive measure in any case) Lanolin creams, such as Lansinoh, soothe sore, cracked nipples and silicone gels offer comfort to sore nipples. See chapter 7 for more on breastfeeding.

Other Issues About the Mother's Body

The new mother may easily overdo it without realizing it. Having a new baby, after all, is exciting but by caring for herself properly, she is likely to regain her strength more quickly. You can advise her about important issues such as fatigue, the appropriate amount of exercise as she recovers her strength after birth, and contraception as she and her partner resume sexual activity (see the section "Sex and Contraception" later in this chapter). A fuller discussion of women's feelings about their own bodies after delivery can be found in chapter 5.

Fatigue

The new mother needs to rest as much as possible, especially during the first week postpartum. Your job is to facilitate that rest by suggesting it and making it possible.

Remind your clients that rest and sleep are not the same thing. They can rest for far more hours than they may sleep. Lying down during the day may seem self-indulgent to today's very active woman. Remind her that these weeks are exceptions to the rest of her life in every way, and she owes it to herself, her baby, her partner, and the rest of her family to take care of herself.

Encourage the new mother to enlist assistance from every member of her household over the age of two. Even a small child can bring a clean diaper or burp cloth to a parent.

Explain to your client that with proper rest and sleep, she can return to normal much more quickly, not that anything truly returns to normal after a baby arrives, she will settle into a new normal. If you find her climbing a ladder or scrubbing floors, reinforce the importance of avoiding heavy work for at least three weeks after birth.

The new mother must learn to trust her body in many ways, just as she did during labor and delivery. Her body will tell her if she is doing too much: She will bleed more or become exhausted and possibly depressed. If she looks very tired, suggest a nap and take over. Remind her, "Listen to your body."

General activity

All new moms should limit stair climbing for the first two weeks. Others can fetch and carry for her, and she can train herself to take what she needs with each trip. Setting up "baby stations" in the areas of her home where she spends most of her time should make most trips unnecessary.

The only problem may be if she spends most of her time on a floor of the house that does not have a bathroom If so, she should consider restricting her time to the floor that does have a bathroom, and allow others to bring her what she needs, at least for the first few days or week after birth.

Exercise

Strenuous exercise should not be attempted for four to six weeks postpartum. The exercises described below and Kegels may usually be started one to three days after a vaginal birth, according to the medical provider's instructions. Daily walks, starting with short distances and gradually increasing in length, can begin about a week after vaginal delivery. Women who have had c-sections generally take longer to rebound and should take it slowly.

Share these simple exercises with mom:

- Abdominal tightening: Lie on your back, knees bent. Take a deep breath. Tighten your abdominal muscles; count to five while exhaling slowly. Release and relax. Repeat four or five times. Do this three times a day.
- Lying on stomach: Empty your bladder. Lie flat on your stomach with a pillow under your head and stomach for half an hour. Do this every morning and night. (It doesn't sound like an exercise, but its good for returning to normal tone.)
- Chin lifts: Lie on your back in bed without a pillow, knees bent. Slowly lift your head until your chin touches your chest. Count to two. Very slowly lower your head back to the bed and relax. Repeat three or four times. Do this three times a day.

Encourage mom to find out about postpartum exercises from their midwives or community. Ask whether she learned simple exercises in her childbirth class that she can start doing shortly after birth.

Many providers supply handouts describing and illustrating exercises. Baby and mom exercise classes, given at places such as the "Y," or stroller exercise classes outdoors, can be fun. As a doula, research and include such local classes in your resource list.

Sex and Contraception

Sexual intercourse is permitted after the stitches have healed, the discharge has stopped, and the mother feels comfortable in the genital area. That usually takes three or four weeks after childbirth. Many doctors advise women not to have intercourse until their six-week examination after birth, but it's a very personal decision and may have less to do with stitches and bleeding than emotions and tiredness.

Consider asking the woman how she feels about resuming sex or see if she brings it up herself. Just be open and available to listen and talk about a topic that's important to her but that she may not be comfortable discussing with anyone else. Assure her that this is a common concern after birth. Validate her feelings about being sore. She should give herself time to be ready which may take weeks or months.

Encourage her to make it clear to her partner if she is not ready for intercourse. Communication about sex, as with parenting and so much else, is critical to maintain and nurture.

Couples can resume sexual activity with many other modes of expression before the mother is ready for intercourse. Holding, kissing, stroking, and just lying down together and talking may be sufficiently intimate for the moment. Loving touch at this special time can keep partners physically close. The baby's demands could possibly interrupt sexual activity for a while anyway. Many books and articles are available on this subject.

Your client may have heard that breastfeeding is a form of contraception. While that is true to an extent, and only when the baby is receiving no other form of food, it must not be relied upon if another pregnancy would be unwelcome so soon. Women can become pregnant only a couple of weeks after giving birth. Therefore, it's important that couples who do not want another pregnancy yet and who are willing to use birth control at all should be prepared to use some form of contraception the first time they have intercourse after the delivery.

Inform mom that love play can stimulate the production of oxytocin, the same natural chemical that causes milk to be ejected from the body. It may be helpful to keep a towel at hand in case some milk spurts out in bed. Feeding the baby before sexual activity will help prevent breast leakage. Hormonal changes may cause the vagina of a breastfeeding mother to feel very dry, using a water soluble lubricant such as K-Y Jelly or Astroglide before intercourse can help.

Condoms with foam are the best form of contraception to use soon after delivery. After six weeks, women can use other barrier methods, such as diaphragms or intrauterine devices (IUDs). Many women who are breastfeeding can use birth control pills containing no estrogen or use the Depo-Provera injection, a progesterone-only contraceptive. The first postpartum visit with the health care provider is a good time to discuss appropriate birth control methods. As a doula, while it is helpful to understand the various options, you would not advise specific types of contraception, but rather guide a mother to talk with her provider about what is best for her.

Meeting the New Mother's Nutritional Needs

Eager as mom may be to lose the "baby weight," this is no time for a restrictive diet. Most women return to their weight before pregnancy within about six months. For now, the new mother should try to stay as well nourished as she was during her pregnancy, especially if she is nursing. This means aiming for three servings of meat, fish, poultry, dairy products, eggs, or other protein, such as beans, each day, plus PLENTY of fluids. The menu should include a variety of fresh fruits and vegetables and whole grains. Fats, sugars, and salt should be limited. To protect mother and baby from toxins, wash all produce well before preparing it and peel waxy foods such as cucumbers, peppers, and apples.

A nursing mother doesn't have to drink milk in order to make milk. In fact, some breastfed infants become colicky when their mothers ingest dairy products. Encourage a healthy diet and remind mom to drink to her thirst. A nursing mom will often feel thirsty as she sits to nurse, offer water as she settles in to feed and suggest keeping a water bottle near her nursing seat. Water is the best source of fluids, but alternating with low-sugar juices and herbal teas is reasonable. A good thirst quencher is seltzer mixed with fruit juice. Milk production itself requires (and uses up) about 500 calories a day, the amount in (for example) a peanut butter sandwich on whole wheat bread and two glasses of skim milk.

While every nursing baby responds differently to the mother's diet, a few general no-nos apply. We know that mom's diet affects the flavor of her milk and sometimes the color of the baby's bowel movements (beets can turn them red) which can be scary if you don't recognize the cause. So food that goes through mom is obviously going through baby, too.

Breast milk takes on the flavor of foods eaten by the mother; that's baby's way of learning his family's cultural tastes. Lots of garlic and other spices will flavor the milk and may disturb a newborns sensitive digestive system though garlic in a mother's diet has shown to increase the duration of baby's nursing. If a taste is unfamiliar to mom, go light. She can concentrate on what she knows she likes, as long as it's healthy. Advise her that she will quickly become attuned to her baby's dietary likes and dislikes and will learn to adjust her diet accordingly, especially when those dislikes lead to a napless day or a sleepless night. On the other hand, it has been noted that women around the world continue to eat the garlic and spices of their usual diet throughout lactation. If mom and baby both like beans, she can eat beans!

Perhaps more important is to avoid foods that have caused allergic reactions such as asthma or eczema in the mother, father, or a sibling. Babies with close relatives who have allergies are more likely than other newborns to develop allergies as well. In such cases, nutritional counseling from a physician, allergist or dietitian would be in order.

You and mom can be reasonable about this. If there is doubt about any food, she should eat small helpings until she finds out whether they affect baby's stomach. It won't take long to learn which foods, if any, distress the baby and should be avoided.

Whatever mom drinks, baby drinks. Many insist that a nursing mother should strictly limit alcohol and preferably avoid it altogether. Some say a small glass of wine or can of beer a day (not too soon before bedtime) won't hurt, while others insist they might. Excess alcohol can also interfere with oxytocin, the natural chemical that controls the ejection of milk.

Mom should strictly limit foods containing caffeine. These include many sodas (they don't have to be brown to have caffeine in them-read the label; Mountain Dew contains more caffeine than Coke, for example) and any form of chocolate as well as caffeinated tea and coffee. Once again, if taking a couple of bites of a chocolate bar every few days will cheer mom's spirits and it doesn't bother the baby, no problem. Decaf tea or coffee should be all right and calming herbal teas are great.

Women who suffer from heartburn should note their symptoms after eating any chocolate, alcohol, coffee, spearmint, peppermint, or high-fat foods. All are thought to increase the symptoms of heartburn.

If mom is distressed about being unable to eat favorite foods, gently remind her that her commitment to breastfeeding will require a certain amount of self-control and self-denial, just for a while, but the tradeoff is well worth the effort, especially if it means getting more sleep because she stayed away from stimulants that would have kept baby awake. Many foods that might disturb the baby aren't particularly good for mom, either.

Important: Just as they did when they were pregnant, lactating women should consult a medical provider before taking any medication at all, whether by prescription or over the counter. Many drugs travel through the breast milk (and placenta). Thomas Hale is the renowned resource on this topic, refer to his book, *"Medications and Mother's Milk,"* and website website.

Light Massage for Mom

For some reason, the importance of a daily dose of touch has been forgotten, but the need remains, powerfully. What's more, touch improves health by suppressing the production of cortisol and other stress hormones so a massage can actually boost immunity from disease.

A researcher named Tiffany Field who has spent many years investigating the effects of touch found that every group, from AIDS patients to geriatric patients to preemies, blossomed with regular massages.

A massage is like a long hug that sends waves of relaxation through your muscles. Not bad for a tired, stressed-out new mom. She can reciprocate for her tired, stressed-out partner. In fact, the baby loves it, too! (See more on infant massage in chapter 8)

Even a five- or ten-minute back rub, hand rub, or foot rub can help relieve tension and feel very relaxing to a new mother who likes to be touched. As a doula, remember that in almost everything you do, some women will love it and some will reject it. Touch is not a positive experience for all women. Their histories may make it difficult to be touched. Penny Simkin's book "*When Survivors Give Birth*" is a tremendous resource for all doulas. Visit Penny's website and watch her YouTube video on The Effects of Childhood Abuse on the Childbearing Woman.

Always ask mom if she would like a massage and if so, whether there are any places you should not touch. Some women dislike foot rubs, for example.

Caution: Don't massage too close to varicose veins; this can bruise the surrounding skin.

Make it clear that you are not a massage therapist and have no professional training in massage (unless of course, you do, in which case, you may package massage services separately from your doula services.) Say that you'll be like a friend giving her a back rub. Even with no professional training, it can feel wonderful. You can also encourage mom and her partner to have a few minutes alone to give each other a short massage while you watch the baby. Massage is a wonderful way for them to be intimate in the first days and weeks before they can resume sexual activity.

You can buy many tools for massage, such as oils and lotions. Ask mom if you may use some. Let her sniff the bottle first. Hand lotion works, too.

Massage oils are available in community shops or by ordering online. The "Happy Massager" (available from Cutting Edge Press; see resource list near the end of this manual) is a small handle with three balls on it Mom will love to have you make broad strokes up and down her back with this little doodad. Consider keeping a Happy Massager and some massage lotion in your doula bag.

Introduce the idea of a massage at a suitable time, not when everyone is running around. For example, after mom has finished nursing and is ready to nap with her baby, ask if she would like a massage as she falls asleep. It works! You can then finish the laundry, cooking, or whatever else you have agreed upon for that day. If your time is up, let yourself out rather than waking her. Tell her in advance that you may do this and will lock the door behind you if she wants. If you haven't had a chance to talk about it before she falls asleep, leave a note saying what time you left and when you will see her next. Manage your time and before leaving, try to settle the baby and help him to sleep if possible, lay the baby is his sleeping place in the mom's room with her, within hearing range or set up the monitor for her to allow her to get a little more rest even once you've departed.

Soothing Music for Relaxation

Consider carrying with you soothing music for relaxation in case your client doesn't have her own. This is a great idea to add to your own playlists to have with you on visits. Many moms have never done this before and don't have any quiet and calming music. If mom would enjoy it, some guided visualizations or progressive relaxation scripts are another valuable addition to your repertoire.

If mom is stressed, ask if she would like you to play soothing music. After it has played for a couple of minutes, ask whether she likes it. If she does, leave it on while she is breastfeeding, lying down, or having a back rub.

If mom asks to borrow hard copies of music or books, use your discretion. Some people prefer not to lend anything, knowing they will lose some of it. Others are so generous that they'll lend anything to anyone. A compromise is probably best. You might say that you will need the resources for your next job. Or say, "You can use it today and tomorrow, but I'll have to take it with me when I leave on Friday."

One way to refuse to lend one of your resources without sounding too negative is to offer to write down the information if she would like to buy a copy, or if mom wants you to go right out and buy it for her, and there is a store not too far away, go ahead. How you spend your doula time is her decision.

Many doulas have a lending library of books, movies, music or even baby carriers. There are online sites and apps to help you input our items and keep track of who you lend them to if you wish.

An Arm Full of Brian

Look at me, Brian?
No, wait love, instead
Measure the morning
And, shhh, I'll not speak.
Sing to the song that
You hear in your head.
Give me the gift of
The curve of your cheek.

Scold a green shamrock,
And laugh at a star,
Frown at the feel of
Two brown apple-cores.
Borrow a butterfly!
Near, son, or far,
Everything's new, Bri—
What wonders there are—
All of them, all of them

  Yours!

 -*Maureen Cannon*

The Twelve F's of Postpartum

By Penny Simkin, CD(DONA), PT

Here is a suggested format for discussing the postpartum period with prospective parents. The "F's" are one way to organize the information and inject a bit of humor to help listeners absorb the points made.

1. Falling in love with the baby

Few parents are prepared for the strong emotional ties they feel toward the baby. Every slight change in expression, every burp or squeak, every cry, every diaper change finds many parents totally engrossed. The first few days or weeks have been compared to a honeymoon (or, as Sheila Kitzinger termed it, "babymoon") for parents and baby-withdrawal from the world, intense preoccupation and deep fascination with each other, profound feelings of love, lack of sleep, and deep contentment.

2. F (Ph)ysical changes

Women undergo many bodily changes in the first few days and weeks postpartum. Doulas should learn aboUl these and be able to discuss them at length with clients. Resources include my book *Pregnancy, Childbirth, and the Newborn: The Complete Guide* and the pamphlet "The First Days After Birth: Care of Mother and Baby" by Jessica Myrabo. *

3. Fatigue

How can we get the message across that parents need to give sleep a high priority:> For impact, I ask each class member (women and partners) how much sleep they usually get when they are functioning well. l then tell them they owe themselves that much sleep every day whether they get it at night or during the day. I point Oul that 8 hours in bed at night, interrupted by two or three 1-hour feedings, does not add up to 8 hours of sleep' I give them a handout at this class: a card that reads, "Fatigue makes EVERYTHING worse." It can be posted on the refrigerator door.

4. Frustration and fussiness

It is frustrating to try to understand the baby and his or her needs, the "fussy baby," the 24-hour-a-day demands of parents, breastfeeding, and the unpredictability of life with the new baby. My advice is to let the baby call the shots. Meeting the baby's needs, as expressed by the baby, is far less frustrating than trying to control the baby.

5. Feeding the baby

This topic deserves an entire class. Since almost all my prenatal students intend to breastfeed, and many plan to work outside the home, breastfeeding and expressing and storing milk are popular topics

6. Fluids and food for mother

I usually suggest that before birth, people plan meals for 2 weeks and do as much of the food shopping in advance as possible Sometimes just knowing what she is going to eat makes the difference between getting a decent meal and not. I also suggest keeping foods available that are quick and nutritious; for example, cottage cheese, fruit, prepared raw vegetables, a turkey that can be "picked," and so on.

To help ensure enough fluids, she fills a 1-quart pitcher with water each day and drinks a glass between meals In addition, she drinks a 10- to 12-ounce glass of liquid in the morning, at noon, and at night. Two quarts of liquid per day are usually sufficient.

7. Figure

A major concern of new mothers is their physical appearance, especially their figures. For most women, the postpartum body is a shock. After pointing out that extra fluid accumulated during pregnancy takes several days to lose, and that her breasts weigh several pounds, I try to be reassuring about gradual weight loss that takes place over a period of several months, especially if a woman is breast feeding and getting some exercise.

8. Feelings

Here I discuss postpartum blues, depression, and the possibility of disappointment wi.th the birth experience. I describe the difference between blues and depression and discuss the possibility of disappointment if labor was not what she expected. I try to point out that disappointment is normal under these circumstances and let the class know that I would like to talk to anyone who feels disappointed, depressed, or unhappy. I relate my personal experiences wi.th postpartum depression as a way to reinforce my desire to be helpful to them. The pamphlet "The New Parent: A Spectrum of Postpartum Adjustment" by Dawn Gruen* is immensely helpful.

9. Father/partner

I try to describe the special deep bond and the new feelings many fathers experience I note the difficulties they often have in balancing these wi.th job demands and personal needs. I point out that his partner cannot make her usual contributions in their relationship. I do acknowledge the stresses on the couples relationship during this time. Patience wi.th each other and wi.th the situation can be encouraged with the promise that life becomes more predictable and easier wi.th time, most of the time.

10. Family and friends

New parents have a real need for company and companionship wi.th other adults, especially those who are close to the parents and who care about the baby. I try to balance that wi.th the need for rest. I suggest that whenever visitors want to come, the mother should ask them to do a favor, such as stopping off at the grocery store or helping wi.th a task or two around the house. "Never turn down an offer of help'"

11. Fertility and sex

Resumption of sexual relations presents a new set of challenges to parents. Perineal tenderness, decreased vaginal lubrication, breast tenderness, preoccupation wi.th the baby, and sleep deprivation may reduce the interest in sex for one or both parents. Patience and kindness toward each other are all-important at this time. The usual information about birth control is also covered.

12. Freedom

I discuss the feelings of being tied down; the now-complex nature of things that used to be easy, such as running out to do an errand; the "magic" of the grocery store or shopping mall when you have been out of touch wi.th the world for a while; and the need to learn to take the baby along to movies, restaurants, camping trips, and most other places, even though it is complicated and time consuming at first.

*Available from Penny Simkin, 1100 23rd Ave. East, Seattle, WA 98112.

CHAPTER 5

EASING POSTPARTUM ADJUSTMENT

In cultures around the world, the postpartum period is considered a sacred time for honoring women. Rituals surround this life-transforming event, which is rightly treated as a rite of passage. During the first six weeks after giving birth, women are expected to think of nothing but taking care of themselves and bonding with their baby. The mother's own mother and other women go in and out of the home, helping with breastfeeding and newborn care and pampering the new mother, attending to her, talking with her, mothering her. Some cultures hold coming-out ceremonies for mother and baby after six weeks to celebrate the baby's formal entry into the community.

Pockets of those warm worldwide traditions do exist here, too. In Rockland County, New York, for example, Hasidic women go to a certain house after delivery. For seven to 10 days, the new mother's "work" in this house is to attend to her own physical needs and those of the baby. Other women deliver meals to the new mother and go to her home to care for her other children and her husband. A postpartum lying-in period such as this permits and encourages the new mother to get to know her baby.

Doulas strive every day to return that gift to women. We provide mentoring and orientation to the new mother in her new job. She turns to her doula with questions, concerns, and fears. Her doula facilitates "matriescence," a term coined by Dana Raphael to mean the state of becoming a mother. The doula shares her knowledge and experience as the new mother greets and takes hold of her role as a mother.

Needs of the Mother

The first-time mother suddenly has powerful new needs.

If she is breastfeeding, she needs to know why nursing is important, how to do it and how often, how to know whether her baby is getting enough milk, and how to pump, store, and use breast milk. Breastfeeding is natural but learned. Early, appropriate and educated support from Day One is a benefit to getting off to smooth start. Mom needs help identifying her baby's cues, understanding the latch of a baby who is eating vs. sucking and learning the sensations of nursing, which should not include pain. With commitment, desire and solid support, most moms can be successful in nursing. Having a supportive partner (as well as the support of anyone in the home) is a key to her breastfeeding success as is confidence. You are doing a mom a great service in providing good resources and in helping build her confidence with truthful acknowledgement of her strengths. You may point out how contented her baby is after nursing or cheer her on as milk dribbles from a sleepy baby's mouth.

The new mother needs to tell her birth story to a caring person. If she is grieving over a cesarean section, an anomaly in the baby, a stillbirth or miscarriage, or some other loss, she needs help in validating and working through those feelings. She needs to enlist her partner in participating in this time of her life so that he understands what she is experiencing, too. A new mother should be permitted to share her birth story as many times as she wants and needs to help integrate that experience.

The new mother needs reassurance about the physical changes she is undergoing. She needs to discuss her body image: the way she feels about her large breasts, expanded waistline, stretch marks, and loose clothing. Tell mom that, "Fullness is fine" and that she can be proud to bear the signs of motherhood.

The new mother needs to be urged to accept her innate mothering abilities. She needs to be told that her raw emotional state is the result of hormones, fatigue, and the profound changes in her life, and will very likely end. If her mood is very low, she may need professional help (see "The down side" later in this chapter).

Changes in the Mother's Relationships

If the new parents live together, the father now has more time to himself than the mother, who may have almost none. Once he returns to work, especially if he has taken a fair amount of time off, she is suddenly left alone to cope. Siblings must adjust to the presence of a demanding new baby. Mom must adjust to having another child in the house or having a child for the first time.

How Sex Changes

Many factors and events can change the way women feel about sex soon after giving birth. Still fatigued from labor and delivery, they get unpredictable, insufficient amounts of sleep that may be disturbed by the baby's cries at any time. Their households and hormones are in turmoil. Older children may hang on their mothers, who in their eyes have turned to the newborn and away from them. Women who have had an episiotomy or cesarean section typically fear that the stitches or incision will make intercourse painful.

With all that going on, many women have no energy for sex soon after delivery. That is just as well, since the recommendation is not to have intercourse for two to six or more weeks anyway (see chapter 4). Vaginal intercourse may be uncomfortable the first few times after delivery, especially in women who have had stitches. Patience and gentleness will be the key.

Once intercourse resumes, women often find it more comfortable at first to assume a position on top. Doing so takes pressure off the stitches. The woman also is in control of penetration that way and can quickly direct the penis away from any painfully sensitive areas. If your client is concerned about resuming sex and wants to talk about it, advise her that it may take time. Closeness and touching need never (and should never) be avoided. Encourage couples to use their imaginations.

Becoming a Mother

It takes three to nine months, on average, for mothers to assume the mantle of motherhood and acquire a maternal role, according to research by Reva Rubin. Full development, she has found, generally occurs in four steps:

- Anticipatory stage ("Mothers should do ... "). This stage, which occurs during pregnancy, is formed from dreams; from books, television, and movies; from conversations and thoughts; and from observing families with infants. During prenatal conversations and visits, the doula helps the mother-to-be frame realistic expectations so that she won't be disappointed later.

- Formal stage ("Mothers must do ... "). Mothers often feel inadequate and rely on professionals to tell them what to do. They are sensitive to comments about the quality of their mothering. Doulas can help by providing simple, consistent suggestions in easily mastered segments. They can also give moms specific positive feedback about their behavior. For example, ask your client, "How does your dream of motherhood differ from reality?" Discuss her answer.

- Informal stage ("Mothers may do ... "). As their self-confidence grows and they spend more time with their babies, mothers feel more comfortable making their own choices. Doulas can introduce alternative forms of behavior and offer various models of good mothers.

- Personal stage ("I do ... "). Over time, mothers decide for themselves how they will mother their children. Their self-definition strengthens. The doula's contributions from the early days postpartum can promote maternal self-confidence that will last for many years.

- Many factors in the mother's current or previous circumstances can cause a delay in acquiring the maternal role. Some examples:

- Her own illness
- The baby's illness
- Early separation from the baby because of either's illness
- Perception that the baby is "difficult" because of colic, crying, difficulty breastfeeding, or other problems
- Lack of social support
- Difficulties with the partner, such as partner absent or uninvolved with the baby
- Low self-confidence and self-esteem
- Negative memories of the pregnancy or birth
- Giving birth as an adolescent
- Being older than most first-time mothers

- Adjusting to motherhood draws on just about every experience a woman has ever had. Consider some negative experiences that a woman may have lived through. As a doula, you may encounter any of these scenarios:

- The mother had a high-risk pregnancy.
- The mother was hospitalized or placed on extended bed rest.
- The mother had a difficult previous birthing experience.
- The mother previously experienced a perinatal loss such as miscarriage, stillbirth, or death soon after delivery, such as with SIDS.
- The mother is experiencing or has experienced physical abuse, such as child abuse from her parents or battering from her partner, or sexual abuse, such as incest or rape.
- The mother is a teenager and suddenly recognizes the loss of freedom that her newborn represents.
- The partner is uninvolved or not on the scene at all.
- The mother isn't sure who the baby's father is.
- Finances or child care are unresolved issues.
- The mother worries about losing her job or wonders how she will be able to afford to care for her baby
- The mother has suffered a recent separation or loss of a loved one.
- The pregnancy was unwanted. Birth control was not used or was used, but failed.
- The mother may have wanted an abortion but was unable to seek one because of religious or other beliefs, financial constraints, late discovery of pregnancy, non-availability of abortion services, or other reasons.
- The mother was pressured by her partner or family to take the pregnancy to term and keep the baby.

Any of these painful experiences may be troubling your client when you walk in the door. Talk with her. Support and comfort her Encourage her to express her feelings. Empathize with and validate those feelings. Assure mom that "unloading" is not the same as complaining.

The Down Side: When Mom is Sad

Birth is one of the many life experiences in which a woman's emotions are profoundly affected as hormonal changes swirl through her body. These feelings go deeper than time and are still not fully understood. Having anticipated unalloyed, immediate happiness, new mothers and their partners may wonder how and why they can feel bad.

Yet many women, often to their great surprise, suffer from sadness after the birth of their babies. That sadness may range from an occasional crying jag to unremitting depression. Lack of support from an extended family may cause new moms to feel isolated and overwhelmed. The feeling of alienation that results confuses and distresses them. New mothers may feel a deep sense of loss without being able to articulate it or know why. If the baby was premature, has anomalies, or is ill, depression may be part of the grieving process but it may also strike without apparent reason. Many couples who suffered infertility are at risk for depression which surprises them since they so greatly desired a baby.

Along with the great gain of the birth, some things have in fact been lost. The pregnancy is over. A woman may miss the feeling of being pregnant and of life within her. No longer is she treated with that particular deference accorded to expectant mothers by family, friends, coworkers, and strangers at the store. Now the baby is getting all the attention. "Could I feel jealous of my own baby?" she asks herself.

Also gone is control over her routine. Just a week or two ago, before the birth, mom might have gone to a movie or shopping or visiting or out to eat or even hopped a plane on impulse. Now it would seem like a spontaneous act to take a shower.

Her lifelong identity is altering daily. If she has taken time off from a job, she hardly knows who she is right now. The self-assurance and confidence she felt at work may have melted into a puddle of incompetence, confusion, and lost identity with no obvious replacement.

Her relationship with her partner has changed dramatically overnight in ways they have not had the time or energy to explore. Most couples are emotionally unprepared for this. They can barely bring themselves to think about it, much less discuss it with each other or anyone else. They may wonder whether they will ever be a couple again and are frightened. (They will, but never in exactly the same way.)

Few families perceive the full extent of a woman's vulnerability after delivery. Friends and family abruptly transfer to the infant the sharp focus they placed on her for almost a year. Women who have come to depend on the emotional and psychological support that they received during pregnancy, support that may have been more extensive or intense than any they received before, feel this loss acutely.

In summary, even when a baby is healthy and the birth went well, the contrast between expectation and reality can be so great that guilt fuels an unnamable disappointment. Mothers whose babies are healthy and normal can't understand why they aren't on a "high" all the time. How can they be sad when they have such a fine, bouncy baby to love?

The Baby Blues

When a woman suddenly feels sad on the third or fourth day after birth, she probably has "the baby blues," sometimes also called "the maternity blues." This condition, which affects about 50% to 75% of women, usually dissipates quickly, lasting for any period from a few hours to a couple of weeks. (Many studies have noted the relative absence of baby blues in cultures that support the new mother.) Symptoms that last longer than a few weeks after delivery may signify postpartum depression (see below).

A woman with baby blues tends to be weepy and irritable, partly as a result of the rapid hormonal changes she is going through and partly as a result of exhaustion. She may feel angry for no reason she can state. She may lose her appetite and lose weight too fast or feel hungry much of the time and gain weight, making her feel even worse. Emotions can change on a dime.

It is counterproductive to tell a new mother, as too many well-meaning people do, that she "should be happy now" or "shouldn't cry" or should "think of the baby, not herself." "Shoulds" have no place in your exchanges with depressed mothers, who already feel bad about the way they feel but are unable to control it. A depressed mother may not be capable of caring for her newborn until her own needs have been met. Do not invoke "God's will." You can't force someone to make a spiritual experience of a depressive illness.

Many mothers have said that the nurturing touch of a doula helps to alleviate that blue feeling. With a caring, knowledgeable helper in her home, the new mom feels less isolated. She gains confidence as she asks numerous questions about baby care and self-care and whether it's "OK" to feel as she does. The doula reassures her that "the blues" are common and will probably go away soon. Rest, nourishment, medical care, help with housework and baby care, and general nurturing can go far toward helping a mother adjust and feel cared for and supported as she becomes a mother and may prevent the blues from becoming a postpartum depression. Studies show that the support of a doula (during birth) diminishes the incidence of postpartum depression.

Nevertheless, if mom is troubled, its also important for her to consult her medical provider and discuss how she feels. Above all, she must not suffer in silence, especially to "protect" others from her negative feelings. Depression is much easier to treat when it is caught early than when it is allowed to progress. Support at this time may be crucial.

Postpartum Depression and Mood Disorders

This common condition, which (according to Depression After Delivery, Inc., and many other sources) affects at least one in 10 new mothers to one degree or another, is considered a real illness, not a phase to wait out, and requires professional help. Yet it is often misdiagnosed or not recognized at all.

The medicalization of birth in hospitals and the routine separation of mother and baby that was once the norm in the United States, interrupting the bonding process, may have contributed to the high incidence of postpartum depression (PPD) in the U.S. Fortunately, homelike birthing suites are becoming increasingly common within hospitals and hospital rules have shifted in favor of rooming-in, skin to skin immediately postpartum and other motherbaby friendly practices. These changes may reinforce bonding and reduce the number of cases of PPD. Only future studies will tell, and PPD is multifaceted and complex, so while these are positive improvements, many factors contribute to postpartum mood disorders. Postpartum mood disorders may include, postpartum anxiety, postpartum obsessive compulsive disorders (OCD) or even post traumatic stress disorder (PTSD) from a difficult birth or what mom perceives as a difficult birth.

For our purposes, we use the term umbrella term PPD to encompass the range of postpartum mood disorders.

Symptoms and risk factors

PPD hits different women at different times after birth and in different ways. It may start within days of delivery or more gradually, months or even a year after birth, or after a woman stops breastfeeding. The time of weaning, especially if weaning takes place precipitously, is a cautionary time when symptoms of PPD may occur.

The chances of developing PPD are greater in women who have been depressed before or who have close relatives who were depressed. Half of women who have had PPD before will have it again with subsequent pregnancies. First-time mothers who are very young or older than the norm seem to be most vulnerable to PPD. Doulas, take note: The incidence of PPD is higher in women who have had negative birth experiences.

Symptoms may include any combination of a wide variety of physical and mental problems that incorporate those of the baby blues but are longer-lasting or more intense. These include sleep disturbances, chronic fatigue, and a lack of interest in sex-hardly unusual in a worn-out brand-new mother, but PPD goes farther than that and can include difficulty eating, poor concentration, and memory loss. More than a little weepy, the mother may find herself crying frequently and uncontrollably. She may fear that she will harm the baby or herself. Expressing such a feeling is a cry for help that should never be ignored.

Women with PPD may have low self-esteem prompted by a poor body image or negative feelings about the pregnancy. Mood swings are common. One day may be fine, followed by a couple of bad days, then calmness again.

Other possible symptoms include a delayed return of menstrual periods, swelling in the hands or feet, hair loss, headaches, backaches, abdominal pain, bowel problems, and lack of energy. The mother may feel no joy in life. She may have trouble producing breast milk. She may feel trapped, guilty, overwhelmed by hopelessness, and unable to fight her despair or to make sense of her feelings.

Despite the name "postpartum depression," depression itself isn't always present. Some women with PPD just feel very anxious or stressed out. They may experience the classic symptoms of a panic attack: intense fear, fast breathing, pounding heartbeat, sweating, a sense of doom, dizziness, and hot or cold flashes. They may either show little interest in the baby or be preoccupied with him, constantly worrying that something is wrong or calling or visiting the doctor again and again despite reassurances that all is well.

Feelings of failure may overwhelm the would-be supermom. After reading all those books during her pregnancy, she may have assumed she'd know how to do everything, including breastfeeding, without help. Doulas know that moms are great with their babies instinctively, but that doesn't mean they can't use a few tips and demonstrations with so much to learn at once. The baby may be colicky or less perfect than expected, and certain aspects of baby care take time to learn. Once mom realizes that help is needed, she may consider herself defeated or lazy. Having a doula at hand to provide guidance, to explain, for example, that mother-infant bonding isn't necessarily instantaneous but may take days or weeks, can resolve some of those concerns right at the start. Doula support can help reduce the associated stress of transitioning to parenthood (or parenthood second or third time around) and normalize the experiences of a new mom.

Causes and Treatment

Many theories have been offered to explain the causes of PPD. They include hormonal imbalances and other biochemical changes, disappointment fueled by unrealistic expectations of parenthood, unresolved issues from childhood, and the often simultaneous stresses brought by the arrival of a new baby, such as a new home or new job.

Treatment of PPD may include individual or couple psychological therapy or counseling and peer support. Excellent organization such as Postpartum Support International (see the resource list at the end of this manual) can refer women to local professionals and support groups and provide literature and other information. Local referrals should be on every doula's resource list and are often available from the couple's prenatal instructor or from the hospital or birthing center where the baby was born.

Medications are available to treat PPD. Whether to take an antidepressant medication is a subject for mom to discuss with her medical provider. If she is breastfeeding, she should discuss this with the prescriber, however she usually will not need to wait until the baby is weaned. La Leche League, local breastfeeding groups, or hospital-based or private lactation consultants may also be consulted for breastfeeding advice, which is sometimes the very thing that helps a mom struggling with PPD.

What Doulas Can Do

As a doula, it's important to discuss postpartum mood disorders with a family prenatally if possible, and provide resources, information and screening tools in advance such as the Edinburgh Postnatal Depression Scale (this is an online tool, there are many pdf versions available online with an quick search) or the Beck Postpartum Depression Predictors Inventories which is available for purchase to be used by clinicians. This preemptory discussion can help to normalize the occurrence if a mother should experience a postpartum mood disorder and it paves the way for discussions when you're in her home after the baby comes. Create a warm and open relationship in which the mom is encouraged to share her feelings with you, a provider, a spouse or someone else who can reach out to get professional help for her.

Know the signs and symptoms of postpartum mood disorders and without mom even needing to be aware, pay attention to signs while you are in her home. If you suspect PPD, advise mom to call her medical provider right away, but even as treatment is sought, many contributing factors are right there in the home, and you can help to alleviate some of them. Offering words of sincere encouragement is always important, many moms won't believe you, so be sure to point out specific things you observe that are positive.

To help moms adjust to their new role peacefully, encourage them to stay in a robe or nightgown for the first week at home, to take the phone off the hook while resting, to limit visitors for the first two weeks and to encourage their partners to nurture both mother and baby. See chapter 2 for more suggestions.

Encourage mom to establish or reinforce a support network of people who can help in any way. Especially important is hands-on support from trusted friends or family members who can take over infant care and give mom a chance to be alone or with her partner. She might join a support group of new moms or enlist friends and neighbors to call briefly every day to see how she is doing. They should be instructed to ask about her, not just the baby.

Studies indicate that breastfeeding mothers with normal hormone levels and good social support adjust more quickly to a maternal role than bottle feeding mothers do and may be at reduced risk of developing PPD. It has been suggested that women at risk for PPD should be encouraged to breastfeed and given the support they need to do so.

There is evidence that increasing a woman's intake of long chain fatty acids, omega 3, can help with depression and mood. Mention this to mom and advise that she discuss any supplements with her midwife or doctor.

Find ways to support the dad or partner in the home as well if mom is struggling with PPD. They need to understand how they can best help but they also must be heard. They have different concerns and needs than their partner and need caring support as well. Open the discussion with dad in person or via other forms of communication (you should have his is a number/email prenatally), provide books targeted at partners and offer reassurance and encouragement that the woman they know will return with good treatment and support. Many partners are confused or intolerant of mom's reactions, it's important that they know that mom can't just "snap out of it" or "pick herself up by the boot-straps" when she is suffering from a postpartum mood disorder.

Additionally, it's also important for doulas to recognize that dads or partners may also experience forms of depression in the postpartum period. Postpartum Men and other online resources can provide you more information to educate yourself on this issue.

Postpartum Psychosis

About one mother in a thousand descends into postpartum psychosis, according to Depression After Delivery, Inc., and other sources. This dangerous condition requires immediate assistance by a health care professional who is experienced in treating it. While you may never come across postpartum psychosis in your career as a doula, you should be alert for it and prepared to swing into action, making sure mom gets help quickly.

The calm, happy woman you saw during your prenatal home visit may bear little resemblance to the new mother with postpartum psychosis. Seven out of 10 women who experience postpartum psychosis have never had a serious mental illness before. The causes of postpartum psychosis are complex and poorly understood. Assure the mother that she did not bring this condition upon herself. Blaming the partner is also a mistake.

Postpartum psychosis tends to begin between the third and fourteenth day after delivery but can extend into the third week or later. At first, symptoms may be the same as those of PPD, but become more severe over time. The mother experiences an extremely altered perception of reality. She may have hallucinations, delusions, or constant thoughts of suicide or hurting the baby or someone else, or she may show a lack of concern for her own or the baby's welfare. Other symptoms can include insomnia, agitation, bizarre or irrational thoughts or behavior, frantic talking in person or on the phone, and bursts of anger or excessive energy.

Hospitalization for intensive psychiatric treatment may be necessary. Group therapy can also be useful for couples who have experienced postpartum psychosis.

Postpartum Depression Resources

Our Bodies, Ourselves: Pregnancy and Birth, The Boston Women's Health Book Collective

This Isn't What I Expected: Overcoming Postpartum Depression, Karen R, Kleiman M.S.W. and Valerie D. Raskin, MD.

Happy Endings, New Beginnings: Navigating Postpartum Disorders, Susan Benjamin Feingold

Postpartum Depression Demystified: An Essential Guide for Understanding and Overcoming the Most Common Complication after Childbirth, Joyce A. Venis RNC RNC, Suzanne McCloskey

Conquering Postpartum Depression: A proven plan for recovery, Ronald Rosenberg, M.D., Deborah Greening, Ph.D., and James Windell, M.A.

The Postpartum Husband: Practical Solutions for living with Postpartum Depression, Karen Kleinman, MSW

Edinburgh Postnatal Depression Scale This is an online tool, there are many pdf versions available online with an quick search

Postpartum Support International (PSI) (formerly Depression After Delivery) is dedicated to helping women suffering from mood and anxiety disorders, including PPD, the most common complication of childbirth. Provides education and support for families affected.

Mass General Hospital's Women's Mental Health Center Based at Massachusetts General Hospital, a site with information on women's health and special attention and focus to maternal health and PPD

Pediatrician's Office

The waiting mothers beam.
The babies, small and bigger,
Some over-dressed, outraged,
Object with noisy vigor
To being beamed upon.
The conversation bounces
From "Yes? How old is yours?"
To "No! How many ounces?"

- Maureen Cannon

CHAPTER 6

APPRECIATING YOUR CLIENTS'
CULTURAL DIVERSITY

By Dr. Karen Salt

Karen Salt is a professor of Caribbean studies at the University of Aberdeen (Scotland) where she teaches courses on race, power, sovereignty, and the environmental inequalities facing marginalized peoples across the planet. She has a keen interest in island eco-aesthetics and the ways that island peoples try to live in balance with and respond to their natural world. She began her journey in women's health teaching childbirth classes before training as a doula. From her days running her own company offering childbirth education and doula services to teens and families receiving AFDC (Aid to Families with Dependent Children) and TANF (Temporary Assistance to Needy Families) to her many duties within national organizations working on midwifery, childbirth, and mother-baby issues, Karen has focused on ameliorating health inequalities, improving women's access to care, and emphasizing the importance of cultural practices within pregnancy, childbirth, and the weeks to months during the postpartum period. She is the author of Baby Tips for New Moms: Breastfeeding *(Perseus),* Pregnancy Tips for Moms to Be *(Perseus), and* A Doula's Guide to Pregnancy, Childbirth, and Motherhood: Wisdom and Advice From a Doula (Da Capo), A Holistic Guide to Embracing Pregnancy, Childbirth, and Motherhood *(Da Capo). Karen has written articles for* Midwifery Today, Childbirth Instructor, *the* Journal of Perinatal Education, *and other publications.*

However well intentioned your doula care and support, you may occasionally experience situations of cultural conflict as you offer your services to a wider community of birthing women. Current statistics show that the U.S. now contains more individuals who are non-white than ever before. As a consequence, your community may be changing. New residents. New customs. New ideas. New practices. If this has not happened to you, it probably will in due time. And as these clients appear, they may bring with them customs and beliefs that differ from yours. Some of those beliefs may not match information about pregnancy and birth that forms the cornerstone of your education and services. Yes, it would be easy to fall back on the mantra that we are all women; but we say much more than that in our service information, our contracts, and in our interactions.

While the prospect of having a cultural conflict with a client may sound daunting and depressing, it can be an eye-opening and welcome experience. Changing the experience from one of conflict to one of growth depends upon your mentality. The more open you are to understanding the wide arc of human experiences, the more centered your practice can be in offering doula services to women of every background. Opening yourself to the possibility of working with clients who have diverse beliefs and backgrounds will enable you to offer services that are appropriate for any family. It will also allow you to practice our long-serving mantra: a doula for every woman.

Being open and present, though, does not mean that you go into situations without knowledge. You should arm yourself about the cultures within your community and seek out information so that you can know and understand the cultural beliefs that affect how, why, and to whom you should direct your attention? To create an atmosphere centered around respect, the responsible doula must learn about others around her.

The following sections are intended to serve as introductions to the complex issue of diversity. While many points address specific groups or characteristics as a whole, each person conceives of those beliefs and expresses them in her own way. We can only learn what someone may believe, then strive to listen to our clients' individual messages. Because culture is a living and breathing thing, it changes, adapts, alters, and merges with other issues and concerns. As such, a woman can be born into one cultural group, yet practice a cultural tradition that has been learned by her family. You will be in the best position if you never assume and always ask your clients about their practices, beliefs, and concerns.

Who we are is shaped by our families, our faith, and our life experiences. This chapter illustrates what has been observed by others and what you may see yourself. As a doula, you must always expect the unexpected.

Beliefs about Childbearing

The U.S. contains thousands of diverse cultural groups. You can't always see diversity or hear it in someone's speech. Differences may be subtle or isolated to certain incidents. Pregnancy and birth seem to bring many cultural beliefs to the fore. Some women believe they must follow "the way" to reduce the chance of the "evil eye" or do things the way their mothers and grandmothers did, without knowing why. Instead of focusing on why cultural beliefs exist, we will examine what they mean to a doula.

Many people explain pregnancy and birth through beliefs about illness and health within the body. How these states are perceived determines what a pregnant mother feels she may and may not do during pregnancy, birth, and the postpartum period.

Many groups believe that a harmonious, healthy state is achieved only by thinking the right thoughts, eating the right balance of foods, and behaving the right way toward others. Some Latino groups believe that a pregnant mother who shows intense anger may be in danger of aborting her baby or even going into premature labor. Because of these potential dangers, such women are encouraged to remain calm and happy during pregnancy.

A number of Latino and Native American groups encourage mothers to be very active during pregnancy. Many Latinas believe that if they stay active, their babies will be small and their labor will be easier.

Among many Native American communities, pregnancy and birth are considered natural, healthy life occurrences. Pregnant mothers are usually urged to continue engaging in normal activities, but active behavior may be unacceptable, especially during labor. Some Asian and Pacific Islander women, for example, would be ashamed to cry out during labor, preferring to show no pain and avoid verbal expression. At the other end of the spectrum are Arabic women, who are often quite verbally expressive during labor. This resonant sound may even be picked up on and shared by the laboring mother's female relatives. What I am describing are cultural traits, not guarantees, about a woman's behavior.

Labor and birth involve a number of cultural issues that influence how and in what manner a laboring mother may interact with those around her. For example, it is extremely important to some Orthodox Jewish women that no men except their husbands view their bodies. Some cover their heads and wear clothing over their arms and legs. Some remain covered throughout labor, choosing to wear long shirts even while the baby is being born. Many of these women seek out female caregivers for pregnancy and birth, including labor support doulas who are sensitive to the ways their religious beliefs affect their choices.

You may encounter mothers who do not want to be touched during labor or postpartum and those who refuse for cultural reasons to be comforted by your bag of labor aids such as hot compresses and massage oils. You may have to be inventive to comfort a mother in such a situation. For example, she may accept a hot drink but refuse a cold one. Be flexible and discuss with her in advance what she would like and would find comforting.

Cultural Influences During the Postpartum Period

A woman's cultural beliefs influence the postpartum period as well. Many Asian and Pacific Islander groups consider that time of life to be fraught with danger. Mothers are encouraged to rest and recuperate, believing that they can become ill if they are active. To prevent illness, women are heated after birth and given hot teas and foods with healing and toning properties. These women are instructed to remain indoors and to avoid cold drafts and cold water for a specific period of time.

Breastfeeding practices are similarly affected by cultural beliefs. In many cases, traditional beliefs strongly support breastfeeding even when contemporary practices embrace bottle feeding. Positive information about traditional nursing beliefs may be more beneficial for diverse mothers than products and brochures that represent only one culture. A good example is the Rosebud Sioux Tribe who live on a reservation in South Dakota. They created a breastfeeding video for their WIC clients that discusses many of the traditional beliefs held within the community. The female elders of the community are shown discussing breastfeeding customs and their traditional purposes with younger mothers. This video is a powerful tool that reminds the younger mothers of their heritage while illustrating the community's support of an age-old practice.

Some Latina women hold beliefs involving the physiology of breastfeeding that may differ from your own. Because these women wholeheartedly believe that colostrum is dangerous for their babies, they will not believe a doula who insists otherwise. In working with such a client, start by trying to understand her tradition. Learn about the people in your community and how they interpret and believe different cultural ideas. Again, finding information from within her culture may enable you to share different perspectives without appearing as if you are offering a dominant or culturally superior point of view.

Another area of potential conflict involves discussions of family planning. Some cultural groups hold strong beliefs about the privacy of sex and the impropriety of talking about family planning except between a mother and her partner. Discussing this topic without this awareness could bring you into conflict with your client. A good way to tackle this situation is to ask your client about the appropriateness of discussing family planning alone or, if she is coupled, with her partner. Of course, this discussion may include other aspects of postpartum adjustments, such as the resumption of intimacy. Tread lightly here as these issues may be difficult to discuss in a mixed sex environment. .

Nutrition may also be a sensitive issue. If you like to discuss food groups or recommend eating certain foods, be aware that your clients may have very different views on what to eat and what not to eat.

Gather information about your clients' beliefs before you attempt to support them. Prepare flexible alternatives to your standard doula support services and be prepared to apply them as the situation arises.

Diversity Surrounds Us

Our culture is far from homogeneous. The U.S. has absorbed and adopted people within its lands who speak a multitude of languages and hold different customs. This may seem like a new phenomenon, but it is not. The U.S. has always been a land that housed multiple cultures. These communities have enriched our multicultural society and continue to do so to this day. The women from these communities may need doula services—and that doula could be you. They bring quandaries for us to accept and work with. All these current and future clients need doula services. One of their doulas may be you.

Readings on Birth and Parenting in Light of Cultural Diversity

Blessed Events: Religion and Home Birth in America, by Pamela E. Klassen

The American Way of Birth, Pamela S. Eakins (Jul 28, 2010)

Harwood, Alan, ed. Ethnicity and Medical Care. Cambridge, Mass., Harvard University Press, 1981.

Culture, Health, and Illness: An Introduction for Health Professionals, 5th ed. Cecil Helman

Promoting Cultural Diversity: Strategies for Health Care Professionals Kathryn H. Kavanagh, Patricia H. Kennedy

Human Sexuality in a World of Diversity (case) (8th Edition) by Spencer A. Rathus, Jeffrey S. Nevid Ph.D. and Lois Fichner-Rathus (Jan 21, 2010)

Birth Traditions & Modern Pregnancy Care (Women's Health and Parenting) by Jacqueline Vincent Priya (May 1992)

A Gift for New Mothers: Traditional Wisdom of Pregnancy, Birth, and Motherhood by Deborah

Jackson (Mar 10, 2005)

Cultural Diversity in Health and Illness (8th Edition), Rachel E. Spector (Aug 18, 2012)

Dim Sum, Bagels, and Grits: A Sourcebook for Multicultural Families by Myra Alperson (Mar 20, 2001) multicultural adoption

Tools to Understand Diversity

How can you learn about those around you?

1. Know your demographics:

As a doula who is committed to working with childbearing women and their families, you must learn to distinguish between individual differences and cultural beliefs. Understanding who you are and whom you will work with is essential to planning your services. This means you must determine the demographics of your clientele before you start working. Read books and articles. Talk to leaders or spokespersons in your community. Attend support groups and city events. Question local midwives, clinics, and doctors about the cultural aspects of their clientele. This is especially important if you have decided to offer your services to a specific community of birthing women.

2. Develop a cultural questionnaire.

One excellent tool to help you understand your clients is a general questionnaire that elicits cultural, social, emotional, and familial information in a respectful way. Send your clients this questionnaire before your initial home visit or take it with you and present it then. Your clients' responses to these questions should help you design your care services to ease any potential cultural conflicts. A sample cultural questionnaire appears at the end of this chapter.

3. Enlist help.

You may occasionally encounter clients whose beliefs strike you as dangerous; for example, promoting the eating of non-food substances such as clay or baking powder. Try to understand the reason behind the custom and work with the mother and her family to find a compromise within their cultural belief system that achieves the same result without introducing the risk of physical harm. If you are uncomfortable doing this, you may want to speak to a traditional attendant (such as a healer, santero/a, medicine woman) in your community who may be able to offer a safer alternative. Ask the mother herself for such a referral.

Navigating Cultural Variations

The profiles in this section summarize characteristics and beliefs observed and identified in childbearing families of four major cultural groups in the United States: African-Americans, Native Americans, Hispanics/Latinos/Latinas, and Asian-Americans. The descriptions of their philosophies and values that follow are unavoidably general and should not be interpreted as cultural guarantees or definitive molds. Every family is different.

African-Americans

History, Past and Present

Most African-Americans are descendants of slaves. Some can trace their lineage beyond Africa to South America, the Caribbean Islands, or Europe. At present, most African-Americans are geographically centered in the South and in large cities. Although this section discusses Americans of African descent, it is worth noting that black Africans, Afro-Caribbeans, Afro-Latinos/a, and black Europeans are different groups that may have completely different cultural beliefs.

Beliefs About Health and Other Issues

Many African Americans view pregnancy as a healthy time. A pregnant woman may have a wide group of family in attendance with her at classes and visits. The term "family" is used loosely. People referred to as "aunt," "cousin," "sister," or "brother" may not be blood relatives, although they are treated as such.

Depending on each woman's faith, it is possible that ministers, pastors, and preachers are held in high esteem. Families may consult religious professionals regarding family issues and problems before seeking help from someone outside the community.

During Pregnancy

Pica, the craving or consumption of non-food substances, including soil and cornstarch, may be part of the mother's diet. This is more true in some geographic locations than in others.

Delaying prenatal care may be consistent with health beliefs, justified largely because the mother is not believed to be at risk prenatally. Many mothers assume that as long as they feel good and the baby is moving, all is well. Due to a variety of issues, including access to care, some women may not see a health care provider for a checkup until the third trimester. Fortunately, this situation is reversing itself. Increasingly, women from a variety of ethnic groups are choosing early and consistent prenatal care.

Postpartum

Many African American women consider the postpartum period to be a time of sickness. Cold air is believed to be responsible for bringing most illnesses. New mothers are encouraged to avoid sudden cold changes and drafts. Restrictions may include the forbidding of tub baths, showering, or washing of hair.

To give the mother time to rest after the birth, other relatives tend to care for the rest of the family. Younger mothers are encouraged to take it easy and to rely on more experienced mothers in the family. Sometimes the result is that others continue to care for the child after the time of rest has ended. If you are working with a young mother, she may be uncertain of her role in her baby's life due to the support network.

Activity restrictions may last for one to two weeks. The mother may avoid cold foods after birth with an eye to seeking heat or warmth for the uterus and other vital organs. The reason is to prevent illness in the mother. Some women omit liver and other meats that they believe cause excessive postpartum bleeding. Again, some of these beliefs may be known, but not practiced and practiced, but not able to be fully articulated as to the reasons why. Talk with your client.

If you are working with a mother who plans to place her baby with another family or receive her baby through such an arrangement, do become versed in the issues of transracial and intra-racial adoption. Many African American communities have strong views on transracial adoption. One reason for discouraging this form of adoption is the desire for African-American babies to stay within African-American families. Learn the mother's feelings. There is a longstanding tradition in the African-American community of informal adoption by blood relatives and non-blood relatives. Formal adoption is often not chosen because a young mother would rather turn her baby over to a grandmother or aunt until she is able to care for the infant herself.

Breastfeeding

In general, southern women tend to breastfeed more than their northern counterparts. There are a number of possible reasons why, including labor concerns. Many mothers have questions about milk production: How much will I make? What can affect it? Some mothers strongly believe that their milk can potentially sour in the breast and make their baby sick. Older women tend to support nursing, especially if they nursed their own children. Again, what a particular woman will believe will depend on the cultural knowledge passed and practiced within her family.

Native Americans

The term Native American refers to a host of tribal groups that reside in the Americas. Many groups prefer to be called by their individual tribal name rather than the term Native American, Native Peoples, or American Indian. Always ask your client what she wishes to be called. For simplicity, this section uses the term "Native American" and summarizes the beliefs of a number of different tribes.

History, Past and Present

In the past, many tribes were clan driven. This social and political structure is still observed by some groups. About 22 % of all Native Americans live on reservations. More than a quarter of Native Americans and Alaskan Natives are under the age of 18.

Beliefs About Health and Other Issues

For Native Americans, health is holistic and reflects living in total harmony with nature. Religious beliefs are interwoven with health maintenance. Many believe that illness is often caused by a spell or a violation of behavioral prescriptions.

Healing care is given by chosen or divine individuals. They are known by a variety of names, such as "medicine women" or "singers." Clan members may refer to relatives by honorific titles. "Grandmother" or "uncle" may be a title of respect given to numerous relatives, depending on whether the tribe is formed by matrilineal or patrilineal descent.

During pregnancy

Pregnant women are usually encouraged to be happy and to think good thoughts. They are frequently urged to eat or avoid certain symbolic foods.

Many communities consider pregnancy a natural event and may not be concerned about whether the mother seeks preventive prenatal care. This has changed somewhat with the urging of the Indian Health Service (IHS) on most reservations to seek such care. Since most Native Americans do not live on reservations, outreach efforts and education beyond reservations are important.

Postpartum

Mothers may be urged to drink herbal teas to tone the body, especially the uterus. Mothers may be encouraged to rest for a prescribed period of time.

Certain tribal ceremonies or rituals may have to be performed by a traditionalist to ensure a good future, a good birth, and a healthy baby

If a baby is to be adopted, a Native American family or relative of the mother is usually chosen as the adoptive parents. Non-native families are rarely given guardianship of a Native American child in place of the tribe or the extended family. Again, this depends on the particular circumstances and practices of the mother.

Breastfeeding

Some mothers may not begin breastfeeding immediately. Many communities believe that breastfed babies think better and have better skin. This belief is usually expressed by mothers who follow the traditional ways of their tribes.

Family planning

Some families have religious or cultural objections to family planning. They may object to discussing sexual relations so soon after birth. A number of communities prohibit sexual contact until the mother is no longer bleeding from the birth or nursing. Some women still rely on herbs and teas to induce pregnancy, aid in birth, and prevent conception.

Hispanics/Latinas

Women who are considered Latina or Hispanic comprise a wide variety of individuals from a wide range of countries in the Americas. Yet some women object to being called by either name and prefer to identify with the country or region where they were born. Always ask your client what she prefers when you discuss her family of origin. Do make sure that you ascertain whether this identification is important to her and why.

History, Past and Present

Mexican-Americans are the largest group of Hispanics/Latinos in the U.S.

Beliefs About Health and Other Issues

As a whole, Hispanics/Latinosh deemphasize time. Time is more fluid and may be determined more by the completion of tasks and projects than by the clock.

Family responsibility dominates, for example, it may be more important to help a family member than to attend a meeting.

Privacy and modesty may be extremely important. Keep overt sexual or visual materials to a minimum. There may be a decision-making hierarchy in which there is a person designated to make important choices for the entire family. Even if you disagree with this structure, you must work within its context in order to support the family.

Home remedies and traditional healers are common. You may find it difficult to ascertain just who these healers are without having prior knowledge of their existence. Some terms in various Hispanic/Latino communities for people who provide healing are santeros, curanderos, partreras, and espiritistas.

Many people believe that health is a sign of rightness and good living. They believe that following certain prescribed ways results in good health. Illness, in contrast, represents an imbalance in the body caused by behavior, punishment, or wrong foods or medications.

Many Hispanic/Latina women groups believe strongly in the four body humors:

- Blood, which is hot and wet;
- Yellow bile, which is hot and dry;
- Phlegm, which is cold and wet; and
- Black bile, which is cold and dry.

For a person to be healthy, these four humors must be in balance. Everything that affects the body including medicine, food, physical manifestations of illness, and biological events such as pregnancy and birth falls into one of these categories.

During pregnancy

Many women believe that physical activity is very important to the size of their baby. They believe that engaging in more movement creates a small baby and, theoretically, an easier delivery.

Some women believe that sexual intercourse during pregnancy lubricates the birth canal, increasing the chances of having an easier birth.

Crying out in pain during labor is encouraged. The mother is usually attended by her mother and perhaps by many members of the extended family as well.

Postpartum

Mothers tend to be advised to stay in bed for at least 30 days. Those who would find this restriction impossible to fulfill may adapt the restriction to fit the family situation.

The mother may be bound around her waist with a faja (cloth) to prevent cold from entering her organs. She may wear a binder to join the abdominal muscles after birth and reduce back pain. Bathing is usually restricted during the time of rest.

Breastfeeding

Nursing mothers are told to be careful of extreme temperatures, both cold and hot. Heat is believed to curdle the milk.

Factors influencing the mother's breastfeeding:

- Her belief or disbelief in throwing away colostrum
- Her belief or disbelief in breastfeeding on or about the third day
- Her belief or disbelief in modesty and privacy issues and possible reluctance to breastfeed in public
- The routine dispersal of baby formula by the staff of the hospital nursery
- Sexual intercourse may be delayed postpartum for a period of time

Asian-Americans

Asia is a huge continent containing a wide array of cultural groups. Beware of applying stereotypes or assumptions about one group onto another group.

History, Past and Present

There are millions of Asian-Americans in the US. The two largest subgroups are from China and Japan.

Beliefs About Health and Other Issues

Most traditional families are male dominated. Many Asian-Americans have a strong belief in the balance of the elements. They feel that this balance must be respected and achieved.

For some, chi is an energy present in all living things. Food becomes chi and has a force that can manifest itself in the body as either yin or yang. The need for balance in one's diet is important.

During Pregnancy

Pregnancy is typically viewed as a natural process. A number of different herbs tend to be used. They are typically dispensed by an herbalist. Certain foods may be avoided during labor.

Many women consider it shameful to cry out in pain during labor. The mother of the birthing woman may be present to provide support during labor.

Marrying and having children at a young age is a traditional cultural value among many Southeast Asian groups.

Postpartum

A balance of the elements is sought. After delivery, the mother and infant may have to be covered to protect them from cold air. The mother may not bathe or shampoo during the postpartum period. She may sincerely fear becoming ill if she permits cold air or water to enter her organs.

For the same reason, she may avoid cold beverages. She may want to achieve the right balance in her food intake by avoiding cold foods altogether after birth. If so, she would most likely consume hot teas and hot soups.

Breastfeeding is traditionally encouraged. Contraceptive information is appropriate to share unless the woman has religious objections to it.

A sample intake cultural questionnaire for mothers

1. Whom do you consider to be a part of your family?

2. Who will be with you during labor?

3. How do people in your community greet each other?

4. How are insults expressed?

5. What behavior by an outsider is considered a sign of respect? Disrespect?

6. What languages do you speak? What language do you speak at home?

7. Do you follow any religion? If so, will this religion affect your labor and birth in any way?

8. How does your family feel about your pregnancy?

9. What activities can a pregnant or new mother do in your family? Not do?

10. What food should a pregnant woman eat? Avoid? How about during labor and after birth?

11. Have you been craving any particular food? Do you eat it?

12. In your family, who is welcome at a birth?

13. Is there any particular person that you would like to have with you at your baby's birth?

14. How does your family tend to respond once a woman has a baby? During the early weeks postpartum?

15. How long, ideally, should a mother rest after giving birth? How long do you plan to rest?

16. Should a mother breastfeed her baby? Do you plan to breastfeed? For how long?

17. Would it be appropriate to talk briefly about sexual relations between you and your partner during our visits?

18. What are your major concerns about labor and birth? After the baby is born?

19. Do you see anyone else in your community for care? If so, what advice or council do they give you? Does your midwife or doctor know that you attend this caregiver?

20. Is there anything else that you would like to tell me that will help me understand you, and if appropriate, your partner?

Developed by Dr. Karen Salt© 1997, 1999, 2013.

When Jamie Smiles

When Jamie smiles, suns leap in skies that shimmer.
Suns dance, and he's encircled by the light
(As we are too) and, oh, we know to him a
Small secret's been revealed, one that he might
Be sharing in a moment-and-a-half's
Sweet time (if we behave). And Jamie laughs!

- Maureen Cannon

CHAPTER 7

SUPPORTING THE BREASTFEEDING MOTHER

This chapter recognizes and appreciates the guidance of Opal Horvat, BA, IBCLC

One of the original postpartum doulas, Opal has many decades of experience with hands on assistance in getting mothers on the path to successful breastfeeding. As well as a former postpartum doula, she has worked as a Lactation Consultant for the WIC Program, training and supervising peer counselors and helping thousands of mothers and babies for twenty years. She has also been a LLL member for 25 years and has breastfed her two sons. Currently she is in private practice and does home visits in Bergen, Hudson, Passaic, and Essex counties in NE New Jersey and Donna Williams, MA.

Donna has decades of experience as a mother of four and now grandmother, too. Donna was an IBCLC, LLL, WIC LC, doula trainer, and in private practice. Inspired by the online learning potential of the first edition of Nurturing Beginnings, *she changed careers and taught technology in an elementary school. She is intrigued to combine these two passions to assist postpartum doulas.*

Often, we have heard from moms, doulas, and medical providers that new breastfeeding mothers need the help of a sympathetic and informed person, someone who will listen to their concerns and offer suggestions. They need encouragement, they need guidance, and they need a friend. They need someone like you.

Women who are lucky enough to have the assistance of a postpartum doula often report later that they breastfed longer and felt an enhanced sense of self as mothers thanks to the information and support their doulas supplied. It is likely that many, or even most, of the women you work with will be nursing, since breastfeeding mothers may tend to seek out the extra support a doula provides. As a postpartum doula, additional and continuing breastfeeding education will serve you and your client well.

This chapter provides basic information that you will give you the start you need to provide effective breastfeeding support. Breastfeeding usually goes well when mom understands what to do right from the start. Postpartum doulas are in an excellent position to get nursing in gear immediately, preventing situations that can cause problems or difficulties, and knowing when to refer to lactation professional.

Encourage the breastfeeding mother to talk with her medical provider whenever she feels she needs to. She should definitely call if she develops a fever or is extremely tired, depressed, or physically uncomfortable when nursing. Urge her to call if she is in doubt whether she should or not.

There are many excellent Internet sources of information on breastfeeding and many local, regional, and national conferences, workshops, and courses for continuing, updated breastfeeding education. The American Academy of Pediatrics Breastfeeding Initiatives site has a section for professionals and for families. Another good source is the mother-to-mother breastfeeding support of La Leche League. By helping women with breastfeeding, you will assist many new mothers in giving their babies a healthy start in life.

Having a few favorite YouTube videos on nursing to show mothers is helpful. Watching a film of a real baby as he takes a couple of tries to latch on and then succeeds can be very reassuring to a new nursing mom. Dr. Jack Newman's website, Breastfeeding Online, is an excellent resource with many videos, pdf handouts and information for moms and professionals. In the children's bookstore section, this site also suggests children's books about breastfeeding, which are great to keep in your doula bag for reading to older siblings. You can observe films of normal newborns nursing during the first week such as how to get a good asymmetrical latch and how to do breast compressions in the early days to keep a sleepy newborn swallowing.

Two blog sites to give you a boost of daily inspiration and humor as you work with new mothers are: Momzelle and for humor, images and inspirations try the Breastfed Blog.

A Doula Speaks

The major goal for a postpartum doula is to find a way in each situation to support and encourage the mom, to help her trust her own knowledge and intuition. She needs to know when to refer to a breastfeeding expert,

Situations you may encounter will run the gamut: from the mom who has had premature twins but can't nurse yet because they're too small, and maybe still in the hospital, so she is pumping her milk to give them in bottles, to the mom who has come home feeling very tired after a cesarean section and is discouraged to the point where she feels that she just can't nurse. You help her find the strength within herself to nurse and do everything possible to create the supportive environment.

An Early Start: Before the Birth

Many woman have pre-set ideas on breastfeeding and will have varying degrees of commitment to initiating breastfeeding. Some mothers will be strongly committed to nursing no matter what struggles or hurdles she faces, others may say, "I'm going to try and see how it goes." All women will need and deserve early, positive support.

Discuss breastfeeding at the prenatal visit. Find out how she feels about the prospect of breastfeeding. If you wait to talk about breastfeeding until after the birth, mom will almost certainly have made her decision already. Although that won't be too late to start if she changes her mind, plant the idea earlier, during her pregnancy. Phrase your inquiry with care. If you ask a yes-or-no question, such as "Do you plan to breastfeed?" and the answer is a blunt "No," your opportunity to present the benefits of breastfeeding may come to a sudden halt. It's better to draw out questions from women who are uncommitted but considering the possibility of nursing. Initiate a real dialog with an open-ended question such as "What are your thoughts about breastfeeding?"

What you hear may surprise you. So many women today have never seen anyone breastfeed that they feel confused and inadequate before they even start. They may be afraid that their breasts are too small to nurse, for example, or that they have the "wrong personality" for it. Listen non-judgmentally to these closely held fears, do not laugh or joke about them, and gently provide reassurance, it's important for doulas to understand commonly held myths about breastfeeding to provide moms with accurate information and guidance. Point out that breastfeeding kept the human race alive for millions of years and "you can do it, too."

If time permits, show the mom-to-be a short breastfeeding video. By watching a good one, such as "Amazing Talents of the Newborn," moms will observe that women were meant to breastfeed and can gain confidence in nursing and enjoy seeing the capabilities of a baby to interact and engage his parents. The breastfeeding portion stars at about 22.5 minutes.

Women who are considering breastfeeding may worry that breastfeeding will "ruin their figures." To them, you may explain that lactation has a minimal effect on the breast once breastfeeding has ended. Rather, nursing can help mom return to her weight before pregnancy. Pregnancy does, however, cause breast changes.

Women may wonder if they'll be "tied down" and never able to go out. On the contrary, breastfeeding is less restrictive than bottle-feeding in many ways. Mom can take the baby anywhere without worrying about keeping a bottle cold and then heating it to the right temperature or carrying around cans of formula. She always has the option of expressing or pumping and refrigerating or freezing milk for someone else to feed to the baby if she can't take him along.

When you are hired, explain to mom what your experience and training are in supporting breastfeeding moms. You can explain and seek permission to discuss any problems you are unfamiliar with or those that may affect her health or her baby's with a lactation consultant or other expert so that you can learn to be more of a help to her. Know when to refer to a lactation consultant and let mom know that this is something you will do if you feel she could use more support and guidance than you are able to provide. Be aware that anyone can call herself a "lactation consultant," but they are most definitely not all the same. An IBCLC, International Board Certified Lactation Consultant, who has been certified by the International Board of Lactation Consultant Examiners, has undergone rigorous education and testing.

Assure mom that any concerns she may share with you about breastfeeding, like anything else she confides to you or that you observe in her home, will remain private. Mothers may be fearful about discussing breastfeeding issues if they believe their comments might be passed along. As discussed in Chapter 1, have families sign a confidentiality form before you begin working together.

Pay attention to the way mom runs her household. Does she have baby gear all over the house or restricted to a single room? Check out potential nursing areas in the bedroom and elsewhere. Perhaps she will want to buy or borrow certain items, such as a footstool or small table, in advance. Many moms like to nurse in a recliner or rocking chair; has she thought about getting one? Chances are that a first-time mom or a first-time breastfeeding mom will not have thought of these things. Help her stock a small basket with things like a phone, burp cloth, magazine, TV remote, water bottle and snacks in her nursing area so she can minimize interruptions once she's settled in to feed her baby.

During or at the end of the prenatal visit, and whether she has said yes or no (unless the "no" was extremely firm), hand your client a pamphlet or two about breastfeeding from one of the major organizations whether you have discussed the issue or not. Say, "Here's some information for you." Open the door to breastfeeding and where she will find resources. Give mom a tangible reminder so that she will really think about it before the birth.

If a woman has flat or inverted (inward-facing) nipples, which are rare, the baby may not be able to latch as easily. Although infants that are with mom skin to skin for the first hour after birth, often surprise us and latch just fine. Also, as the breasts enlarge during pregnancy, inverted nipples tend to "pop out" naturally. Women with inverted nipples may need extra patience. Nipple everters, devices that consist of a syringe with a soft, flexible silicone tip that gently pulls the nipple outward for easier latch-on are available for purchase online, at baby stores and through lactation consultants. Other ways to reverse inverted nipples are with breast shells or an electric breast pump. Women with inverted nipples should discuss what to do with a lactation consultant or medical provider, preferably during pregnancy.

Some Benefits of Breastfeeding

Nursing provides a unique bond with the baby and medical science supports it too. In February 2012, the American Academy of Pediatrics reaffirmed its breastfeeding guidelines: " AAP reaffirms its recommendation of exclusive breastfeeding for about the first six months of a baby's life, followed by breastfeeding in combination with the introduction of complementary foods until at least 12 months of age, and continuation of breastfeeding for as long as mutually desired by mother and baby." Read the report.

Some women want to be talked into breastfeeding or to learn more. To the hesitating mom, you might say, "You don't need to decide now. The colostrum that comes out after the birth is so good for your baby that you will provide benefits even if you nurse for only the first few days. We call colostrum 'liquid gold' because it's concentrated and supercharged to help your baby with antibodies and immunities." It's easier to stop breastfeeding than to start after a week or more, although that too is possible; even adoptive mothers have done it, with special techniques and tremendous dedication.

Recognition of the dozens of advantages of breastfeeding to mother and baby grows steadily as science attempts to keep up with the mother knowledge of thousands of years. New discoveries continue to bolster the foundation of medical literature supporting breastfeeding with more evidence of physical, emotional, and psychological benefits to mother, baby, or both.

Help moms realize that breastfeeding is the optimal way for women to feed their babies. Keep at your fingertips good resources and referrals for breastfeeding. Kelly Mom is a good resource for moms and doulas and provides links to professional position statements, links to comprehensive lists of benefits, links to medical benefits, and links to studies and information on specific benefits. You can also download the American Dietetic Association's article Promoting and Supporting Breastfeeding.

Women who fully intend to breastfeed appreciate hearing all this, too. Moments of difficulty may come in the middle of the night when mom considers giving up and remembering the many benefits of breastfeeding may bolster her and reinforce her decision to continue nursing.

Many people are swayed by the lure of advertising. The word "formula" may sound scientific, but is more accurately described as "artificial baby milk." It is not the same as breast milk and not the same for the baby. The World Health Organization (WHO) and United Nations Children's Fun (UNICEF) have addressed the way formula companies market their products in the International Code of Marketing of Breastmilk Substitutes.

Ads can be highly effective in subtle ways. Ads talk about "when you stop nursing" and "when you have problems" as though those eventualities are inevitable. These are the messages that register with many susceptible prospective parents. You may have to help them get over any initial negative impressions about breastfeeding.

If it is occasionally difficult, mom should remember that the entire period of nursing is not long in comparison with the length of life. Note to prospective moms who are concerned about being "tied down" that the frequency of nursing decreases tremendously over time. Some newborns want to nurse almost all the time, because breast milk is so easily digested, but even after two or three months they will be feeding at less frequent intervals. Breast milk is always clean, fresh, at the right temperature, and goes with you everywhere. Breastfeeding comes from the heart. Until a woman has nursed her baby, she can't imagine how it feels.

Some Benefits to the Parents

Women like breastfeeding because it's healthier and just plain easier in general. They appreciate not having to deal with bottles in the middle of the night, not worrying about running out of supplies, and being able to put a diaper in a pocket and walk out the door instead of packing and lugging a bag full of bottles and formula.

The physical contact between a nursing mother and her infant enhances bonding. Hormones released during breastfeeding often have a calming effect on the mother. Breastfeeding burns calories, helping mom return more quickly to her weight before pregnancy. Nursing requires no cash outlay, a big boost in difficult economic times. Moms may be surprised to hear that with the money they will save, they can buy a major appliance or stash some cash for the baby's college education. Breastfeeding families have less washing up to do, less garbage to throw out, and less recycling of cans, bottles, and boxes.

Breastfeeding helps the uterus shrink after birth and return to its normal size more quickly. Explain to the nursing mother that her uterine contractions, which feel like cramps, are normal and will help her body resume its former shape. These last only a few days.

Nursing reduces the chances of developing ovarian cancer and breast cancer and builds bone strength to protect against osteoporosis. The longer a woman breastfeeds, the greater the benefits to her and her baby and the longer they will last.

Some Benefits to the Baby

Breastfeeding provides the baby with significant emotional and psychological benefits as well as many boosts to both short-term and long-term health. Each mother's milk is made for her baby, is more easily digested than formula and contains the perfect proteins and nutrients for optimal brain growth.

Bringing immunologic advantages, breast milk helps fight infection in newborns and decreases the likelihood that they will develop jaundice. Feeding the baby nothing but breast milk for at least the first six months of life may prevent allergies to cow's milk and other foods or may reduce their effects.

According to the American Academy of Pediatrics, research suggests that breastfeeding is one of the factors that may help protect against sudden infant death syndrome (SIDS).

Nursing improves peripheral vision, which will be important when the baby is old enough to drive a car, play basketball, or just cross the street. Throughout their lives, breastfed babies have a lower incidence of uterine cancer, ear infections, pneumonia, meningitis, celiac disease and osteoporosis than bottle fed babies do. Breastfeeding may help regulate cholesterol levels later in life.

Studies have shown that nursing raises a baby's I.Q. Breastfed babies' bowel movements smell less offensive than those of formula-fed babies, a situation that is more pleasant for all diaper changers. We could go on and on.

Gee Whiz Facts on Breastfeeding

Some Risks of Not Exclusively Breastfeeding

Breastfeeding has many benefits. Besides the fact that it is always the right temperature, clean and ready, breastmilk contains at least 200 more nutrients than formula and it is protective. One list of the risks of not exclusively breastfeeding for the first 6 months (at which time solids are introduced and included) from the Pulaski County Health Dept. includes: "60% more likely to suffer from ear infections, 40% more likely to get diabetes, and 30% more likely to suffer from leukemia." As the knowledge of these risks are becoming part of the fabric of our culture, more and more mothers are determined to breastfeed. They need all the support that they can get.

Who Needs Help?

The answer is any woman is likely to appreciate your counsel and assistance with breast-feeding. Women who want postpartum doulas do tend to breastfeed and to expect their doulas to aid them in their efforts. Even if mom is doing great and you are basically a cheerleader, that may be enough. She really needs to hear your praise and will bloom under its glow. Confidence is key for the breastfeeding mother.

The women who are nervous about nursing have often heard or read negative comments and anticipate problems. Let them know that most women do just fine, and any problems that may arise can be managed by referrals to local professionals who can provide more intensive, specialized care.

Many women who seemed confident when their mothers or grandmothers were staying with them after the birth find that they want more breastfeeding support when their relatives leave. Other times, grandma never nursed or hasn't nursed in decades, and often can't provide the specific help a mother needs. Mothers of twins or triplets are more likely than mothers of singletons (single births) to say they need breastfeeding help. There are far more multiple births these days as the result of a vastly increased use of fertility drugs and related technology. Women who have premature babies, especially twins, often need help breastfeeding, especially at first.

Your Role as a Doula

Sheila Kitzinger calls the early weeks with a new baby a "babymoon." It takes time for mother and baby to get to know one another. Each baby is different, whether the first or the sixth in a family. During this time, it is best for the mother to spend as much time as possible with the baby and to nurse frequently so that she can establish a good milk supply. She needs support and care so that she can focus on her baby and recover from the birth.

Mom may have to work through some surprise or disappointment about the birth or the baby before she can focus on breastfeeding. Talk it through so that she can help reconcile her birth with her expectations or her reality. You'll find more on this in previous chapters, particularly the section "Integrating the Birth Experience" in chapter 2 and Penny Simkin's essay "A day you'll never forget: The day you give birth to your first child."

Prenatally, suggest or loan her some books related to breastfeeding. The Womanly art of Breastfeeding is in its eighth edition and very reader friendly. Recommend some websites such as Breast Feeding Online to read about latch, breast compression and other breastfeeding skills or watch videos online - Baby-Led .

Your presence as a doula will help the new mother begin breastfeeding and enjoy it while keeping housework and outside pressures to a minimum. Compliment her successes and act quickly to correct situations that can create problems, such as poor positioning. Getting additional training, taking professional development courses, online continuing education and having experience in how to help a new mother with nursing will be valuable as a postpartum doula.

Help mom to get plenty of rest and drink fluids. Give her the kind of support that she needs but might not give herself. Before each nursing session, get mom comfortable and relaxed. Read about proper positioning later in this chapter and watch her closely, rearranging pillows and making her comfortable as needed. Bring her a snack and a diaper or clean cloth for spit-ups..

Observe the setting and mom's personality. Would it be helpful to draw the curtains during nursing sessions so that people won't see in the window? Can you move a small table for food and a drink next to her "nursing station" so that she can sip and eat while nursing? This snack is a good habit to initiate so that she routinely drinks, eats healthfully and cares for herself.

Should a floor lamp or table lamp be moved closer to the bed or chair so that she can reach it to turn it off if the light shines in the baby's eyes? Can you find a large blanket or quilt to put around her shoulders and the baby on cold nights? Is a basket of toys nearby for older children to play with while the baby nurses?

Can phones be turned off during nursing sessions, and would mom like that? Would she prefer music or silence as she nurses? If she has short legs, would she benefit from having a footstool or a pile of book on the floor in front of her chair? Think ahead, anticipate and suggest things that may make her more comfortable. Now you're really a doula!

If mom would like to watch TV, place a remote near her nursing chair. Nursing will have to fit in with her lifestyle. Assess this and help her to work with it.

While nursing, mom may want you to sit with her and admire her prowess. Offer constant praise and reassurance. New moms are sensitive. They may think the baby "doesn't love me" if he won't latch on right away. Point out that babies are tense when they are hungry and relaxed after a feeding. Say, "See how the baby likes you and is looking to you for his meal. He knows just where to go."

Babies may smile at the end of a feeding; if so, point this out or note how content the baby looks, sleeping now in her lap. Give her extra doses of confidence and support that will help her persevere.

If mom is happy on her own, nursing sessions can be good times for you to accomplish other tasks. You might quickly check on a meal you are cooking or change the sheets so that mom can climb back into a clean bed when the baby is done. You can read a story or children's book - perhaps one about breastfeeding - to an older sibling, who may feel left out during that special nursing time.

For moms who have not started to breastfeed but seem as though they might want to, encourage her to contact a lactation consultant, as early professional support will help get a mother off to a good start, even after a delay. Talk with mom's partner, whose help will be needed for her to continue. A partner's support is shown to be one of the single greatest factors in a mom's breastfeeding success.

Be a good influence to those who will give your client support after you have left. Mom's mother, mother-in-law, grandmother, or friends may react to her decision to breastfeed in unexpected ways. If those of older generations were discouraged from breastfeeding their own babies, they may be bewildered by society's complete turnaround and jealous at having missed the experience. They may not be knowledgeable about breastfeeding and may genuinely worry about a variety of things, such as the baby's almost continuous wish to feed. You can help educate and reassure family members and friends so that when you leave the family's home, they will encourage and support her rather than making comments that could discourage her. Call the local La Leche League group. Collect information about upcoming meetings and share it with mom. She may want to go but not have the time or energy even to make that phone call. Encourage her to become a member too.

If a lactation consultant is needed, ask mom if she would like to arrange the first visit while you are there. Most lactation consultants are happy when the doula is present so that the doula can take notes and help remind mom about instructions later.

If it's your style, one idea is to create certificates of achievement with personalized statements such as "Congratulations! You have passed the first week of parenthood" or "Your baby has gained her first pound on breast milk." Present to mom on the appropriate day

Photograph the nursing mother, the one baby picture that people rarely think to take. With her permission, put the picture on a magnet that announces your name and phone number. When mom's friends see it on the refrigerator, they will ooh and aah and it will be a good marketing tool for you, too. Add a message, and your name, or try picture frame magnets with a pop-out center for your name and phone number.

Useful handouts, pdfs and other breastfeeding resources can be found free (Dr. Jack Newman's site has many handouts) online as well as many for purchase. The Healthy Children Project offers books, movies, pamphlets; tear off pads and other materials. The Womanly Art of Breastfeeding Book has a tear sheet toolkit in the back which are also available online.

How the Partner Can Help

The attitude and actions of the dad or other partner can be an important factor in determining whether mom continues to breastfeed or not influenced their decision to breastfeed or continue breastfeeding.

Fathers can discourage breastfeeding if they feel left out, uncomfortable, or embarrassed, harbor medical misinformation, or are reacting to bad advice from others. Men tend to jump in and fix problems. If mom starts to cry or complains that breastfeeding is difficult, dad may want to repair the situation by giving the baby a bottle.

If mom's partner is around when you are in the home, educate him about the endless advantages of breastfeeding and validate mom's decision and desire to nurse. When a mom is really committed to breastfeeding but her partner is not as supportive, overhearing positive encouragement from a doula can help. Subtly, you are modeling supportive actions and words. If you're able to give positioning or hold tips that dads can remind moms of, it helps satisfy their need to do something.

Show him how he can participate, even without breasts. Teach him all the things he can do to help: prepare a drink or snack, get the wipe-up diaper and pillows ready, bring the baby to mom, massage her shoulders, put his arm around her as she nurses and talk to her, encourage her verbally, keep her company. Explain that relaxing her shoulders and relieving nervousness and tension will actually help the milk come down.

Nursing time can be a quiet time for the parents to be together as a couple while enjoying their beautiful new baby. This time with the three of them together allows the new family to bond and get to know each other. Just being there with her is a huge support for the mother. If the baby needs a diaper change after the feeding, dad can be the official changer. Dad can also do the same things you do while mom nurses: change the bed, check on dinner, run errands, tidy up, and play with the older children. All this will make it easier for mom to nurse.

Men love skin-to-skin contact with babies, and their babies love it, too. This act is especially important for preemies (see the discussion of "kangaroo care" under the section "The Premature Infant" later in this chapter). Dads can enjoy this contact whether mom is nursing or not. One dad was dubious about this, but agreed to place his infant daughter on his bare chest as he lay back on the sofa to watch a ballgame on television. When she fell asleep there, he was captivated.

For much more on ways to be a doula to the dad or other partner, see chapter 9.

Draw on Your Own Experience

If you breastfed your own baby, think back about how it felt. On a continuum of 0 to 10, with 10 representing the best possible experience, what number would you assign to yours? What were the highlights? Did anything go wrong? How did you resolve it? Think through these issues for each baby you nursed. Whether consciously or not, you will take your experiences with you to every breastfeeding mother you serve.

Any negative experiences that you (or women you know) may have had can enrich your ability to help others. Sometimes a doula who nursed a preemie or suffered from a breast infection can be more helpful and compassionate with nursing moms who are having problems than a woman whose breastfeeding went perfectly from Day One.

Be careful, though, not to use your personal experience as a replacement for training on how to practically help nursing mothers and guard against projecting your experience onto other women. Each woman, each baby is unique. Breastfeeding, while natural and normal, is a learned skill and requires a learning curve for both mom and baby; some new moms pick it up easily while others struggle and require more intensive support. Simply because someone was successful in nursing her own baby does not necessarily qualify her to adequately offer suggestions and guidance on nursing techniques. Professional training on how to support a mom and an understanding the mechanisms of breastfeeding will build a doula's expertise and confidence in supporting nursing mothers.

The second or third time around, things often are smoother. In breastfeeding as in other aspects of life, we learn from experience and have the confidence to deal with whatever the subsequent baby needs.

Questions Nursing Mothers Ask

Most new nursing mothers need to be reassured that all is normal and they are doing a great job. Keep reminding mom about the benefits that both she and her baby are deriving from this relationship, now and for the future. Comment frequently about how beautifully the baby is latching on, what a lovely picture they make as mother and infant, or any other remark you can think of that is both positive and honest.

If mom is still working on latching-on and nursing hasn't been streamlined yet, you can always comment on how much the baby loves her milk and how happy they will be once everything is coordinated.

Be prepared to answer these questions, which new moms often ask about breastfeeding:

- Is this a good position?
- Is it OK that nursing hurts sometimes?
- Will this baby ever go longer than two hours without a meal?
- I feel as if I can't do anything else but nurse. The whole day goes by and I'm still sitting on the couch, nursing. Is this normal?

Since your role will be to help mom get through the transitional phase of the first few weeks, that's what you should concentrate on. If mom wants to know about weaning, solid foods, or how to continue breastfeeding after the baby starts to crawl, explain that she can get that information when she needs it; there's plenty to learn for now. Giving her a resource list which includes La Leche League or Lamaze will amply demonstrate that resources will be available for each step as she and her baby approach it. Local nursing support groups at hospitals or lactation consultants' offices as well as other new moms groups should be on your resource list as well.

"Why does it hurt?" After the first few days, breastfeeding may involve some tenderness but should not hurt severely or continuously. A nursing mom who feels real pain should contact a lactation consultant, medical provider, or La Leche League leader. The most common cause of pain is poor latch, which can be corrected with proper guidance.

If mom says, "I don't have any milk," show her how to hand express. Show her how to place finger and thumb across from each other about two inches behind the nipple. Push back towards the chest wall and then roll them towards the nipple. Repeat several times; reposition to another push point and repeat, eventually circling around the breast. Demonstrate that there is indeed milk in there. She and the baby just have to learn how to get it out. Manual expression also serves to increase supply as the breast massage increases prolactin, the milk production hormone.

"What if I leak?" Commercially available nursing pads, reusable or disposable are available. Clean, soft handkerchiefs folded into a square and placed inside the nursing bra is another quick option. Mom should change these often and dispose of them or wash them promptly. Plastic-lined pads are not recommended because they lock out air, which is needed to keep the nipples soft, supple, and healthy.

"Should I start pumping milk right away?" Tell mom the best way to get started is to nurse frequently to help baby really learn how to breastfeed. Once baby has it down in a while, she can think about pumping if she wants or needs to. Starting bottles too soon can confuse the baby and cause him to prefer a bottle nipple, so it's best to solidly establish nursing before introducing artificial nipples. Suggest introducing a bottle at about four to six weeks if mother is going back to work. If she waits too long, the baby may reject the bottle. If she starts too early, the baby may start struggling with breastfeeding.

"Can I use a pacifier?" Pacifiers remain a sticky issue. Some authorities say they reduce the length of breastfeeding. Advise mom to discuss the subject with her pediatrician, read about it, and make her own decision. If mom is stuck in a traffic jam and the baby is screaming, using a pacifier won't be the end of the world, but it's best to hold off at the beginning, then reevaluate the situation later. For the first few weeks, the baby is learning to breastfeed, the recommendation is to wait at least one month while nursing and mom's milk supply are established. If you throw in something else, it probably won't help him and may confuse him, interfering with his "breastfeeding education."

Some Advice for Giving Advice on Breastfeeding

You won't go wrong if you follow these guidelines:

Be honest. Explain from the beginning that you are not a breastfeeding expert or a lactation consultant, although such people are available to be contacted if needed.

Listen. When mom expresses her concerns and asks questions, listen closely. Ask questions in return that will help her to clarify what she believes and needs to know.

Remember. If you have breastfed, trust your own experiences, both good and bad, in conjunction with what you have learned as a doula for helping others.

Share. Mom is likely to feel more comfortable asking you for assistance or advice once she senses that you are comfortable with helping her and eager to do so. Nursing moms tend to feel an immediate bond with each other. If you have breastfed, your strongest tie to the new mother may be your breastfeeding history. While moms want to be taught the facts about breastfeeding, most also appreciate hearing helpful hints based on your own experiences as a mother and doula. Begin sentences with expressions like, "Many moms find that...."

Preserve confidentiality. Let the new mother know that any concerns she may share with you about her breastfeeding experiences will remain confidential, and then respect that promise. Most mothers worry about sharing their concerns if they suspect that the information may be discussed elsewhere.

Accepting Differences

Each mother you counsel has had a unique set of life experiences. Even the reasons that women choose to breastfeed are different.

Mothers who want breastfeeding support come from the full range of cultural, religious, economic, and ethnic groups. Their ages and the makeup of their families also vary tremendously. What they have in common is a sincere desire to breastfeed their babies. Focus on the similarities among all nursing mothers and babies while keeping cultural and other differences in mind, as discussed in chapter 6. Your role as a doula is to offer breastfeeding information and support without making judgments.

Educate yourself about breastfeeding traditions in different cultures and always ask families if there are any cultural or religious traditions that you should know about in order to honor and respect them.

Unless money is not an issue for mom, make useful suggestions and choices for purchasing breast-feeding supplies, for instance she doesn't need a sterilizer. Babies can be expensive! Providing for the needs of a new baby may consume any spendable income that a family may have. People can make do without fancy equipment if you show them other ways. For nursing, all a mom really needs is her breasts, a couple of pillows, and a clean diaper or towel for spills.

As a doula, appreciate any practices of the mother and her family with which you may be unfamiliar, whether or not you understand or agree with them. Following practices that have been passed down through her family may be more important to a mother emotionally (even if only to please her own mother) than practical suggestions that you may offer for changing them. It's a doulas role to support and respect a family in the way they wish to parent.

If mom wishes to follow folk practices, don't make a fuss or negative remarks. Do ask about them for your own education. Let her continue unless you are sure a practice will harm the baby. If a certain practice helps her to feel more comfortable, following it will encourage her to continue breastfeeding. For example, if mom's breasts become engorged, explain the standard recommendations for relieving engorgement. If she is trying something else that is safe but not scientific, offer your methods as additional ways, not substitutes, to reduce her discomfort. It is often helpful to present suggestions to moms as something to consider versus something she should do. You are offering tools, options, tips and tricks from your experience and training from which a family may pick and choose what to use and what to reject.

Safety is the only area in which a doula may more definitively state a should or should not, for example, it is important to advise a family that it's unsafe to leave a baby unattended on a couch, changing table, other surface or in the tub.

Keep in mind that not all women have partners (husbands, boyfriends, companions) or family members who are willing to help or even interested in their breastfeeding efforts.. Help her with sources of support to tap after you leave and offer a variety of suggestion from which she can choose her favorites.

Telling a single mom with other young children to "get plenty of rest" will only make her laugh.

Instead, you might advise:

- Enjoy breastfeeding. It may be your only time to sit down.
- Take advantage of any time you can take a break to rest instead of doing housework. Give the children something to do, preferably all in one room, so that you can keep an eye on them and have a little quiet time or do something while sitting down.
- Pick a time when you and the children can lie down and rest, even if you don't all sleep.
- When you feel tired, nurse the baby while lying down.

Skin-to-Skin Beginnings

Pregnancy boosts the body's production of a hormone called prolactin, which stimulates the production of milk in the cells of the breasts that do this job. Breastfeeding further promotes the production of prolactin which is why frequent nursing causes mom to make more milk. Skin-to-skin time also raises prolactin levels and therefore milk production. Prolactin is often called "the mothering hormone" as it relaxes the mother as well.

Lactation, the production of breast milk, begins immediately after delivery when the placenta detaches and is delivered. The first breastfeeding experience should take place in the first hour after birth. Mom should know what to expect after delivery and should be encouraged to ask to hold the baby skin-to-skin for at least an hour, undisturbed. Chest to chest, baby will feel safe as his skin relays that message to the brain. He'll notice her heartbeat in his ear and he'll pick up the rhythm of breathing from her. He'll be warmed and his blood sugar regulated. After a while he'll lift his head and look at his parents. Parents are awed looking into their baby's clear eyes. That "seals the deal"! Within 45 minutes he will start rooting and with a little help from mom, he will breastfeed. The baby will instinctually make his way to mom's breast, will play and lick her nipple and will eventually self-attach. Baby-led breastfeeding is ideal and the baby will get the biggest feeding he will have for the next 2 days - while he is so very alert. All procedures can be delayed so there is no separation if there is no medical emergency.

Kangaroo care is a wonderful way to help the mother and baby bond and to help insure the infant's well-being. Dr. Nils Bergman, MD has been doing research on the neurological effect of skin-to-skin contact (SSC). He is a neuroscientist and neo-natologist in South Africa and speaks at conferences all over the world. His research discovered much more. When baby is skin-to-skin, his vitals are being stabilized as well as SSC is regulating his autonomic nervous system.

During the baby's "journey" to the breast, touch, smell and taste activate nerve pathways that lead to the baby's amygdala. The amygdala part of the brain is the place of emotional memory. Also the baby's limbic system is stimulated, helping to regulate his autonomic nervous system. Bergman calls it "firing and wiring the brain." In this process of sensory stimulation

"Heart rate, breathing and oxygen saturation, blood pressure and temperature all stabilize far faster on mum than when they are separated. Baby has his basic needs for warmth, food and protection met."

Encourage moms to let baby have a good long rest from time to time - upright on her chest with SSC (diaper only). He could be under her shirt with his head out of the top of the shirt. A plain V-neck or scoop neck tee works well. Snug is good.

The milk ejection reflex (MER), or letdown reflex, which happens every time a woman nurses, is triggered by a hormone called oxytocin. The release of oxytocin tells small muscle cells inside both breasts to contract and send milk through the milk ducts. The letdown reflex may be triggered when the mother thinks about her baby, whether the baby and mother are in the same place and whether the baby is crying for food or not. Establishing the letdown reflex is important to successful lactation. It can feel like a tingling in the breast. Many moms report not feeling any sensation, which does not mean she is not having a letdown. Breastfeeding women often feel hungry, thirsty, or "spacey" as the oxytocin is released.

For about the first week, the uterus may cramp during letdown because oxytocin, the same hormone that is stimulating the flow of milk, causes the muscles of the uterus to contract. Tell mom that this is "good pain" because it indicates two things: the uterus is shrinking back to its original size and breast-feeding is proceeding well.

The first milk that emerges after delivery is colostrum, a thick, rich food often called liquid gold that all babies deserve to receive. After three or four days, the consistency of the milk becomes thinner, more like skim milk and sometimes with a bluish tinge

Nursing Positions for Mom and Baby

If baby is well positioned, mom and baby will avoid many potential problems. The doula doesn't have to know how to solve every breastfeeding problem, but this one is important and comes up all the time. Good positioning can make the entire breastfeeding period a more comfortable experience. If positioning and latch is difficult, or if it is painful for more than a minute, or if there is nipple damage, or if the baby is not gaining well refer the mother to an IBCLC.

Your most helpful resources include: Suzanne Colson's website, book and movie of her approach to positioning of Biological Nurturing for Laid Back Breastfeeding, "Baby-Led Breastfeeding and The Mother Baby Dance by Dr. Christina Smillie, is another resource for positioning. In addition, here is the webpage copy of the tear sheet from the Womanly Art of Breastfeeding covering laid back breast-feeding guidelines. You can print this as a handy reference for your moms. Scroll down the page for an illustration and suggestions for laid back breastfeeding or use the pdf tear sheet alone.

The baby should start with his nose to the nipple. Remember that phrase and repeat it to mom often: Start with the nose to the nipple. Mom then holds the baby so that he is coming from below and up toward the nipple rather than straight on. This is called asymmetrical latch. If the baby's head is tilted too far back, too far forward or turned to the side, he can't swallow easily. Try it - neither can you!

Suggest taking baby's clothes off (everything except the diaper) so he can be skin-to-skin in those early weeks. If he is laid on his mother's chest he will calm, listen to her heartbeat for a minute and then show that he is ready by rooting. Mom helps him (no rush) to get nose-to-nipple. If he is at her left breast, she can comfortably wrap her left arm around him with her hand firmly on his diaper support-ing him. One of his feet or knees will probably be between her legs and the other over her opposite leg. The natural position is diagonal. (Rarely is this a problem for a C/sec mom.) Because mom is leaning back comfortably, baby's weight is mostly on her torso. He probably doesn't feel heavy, but if he does - a pillow can support her elbow

A mom should support her baby's head from behind his ears with the heel of her hand between the baby's shoulder blades instead of holding the baby by his head. Trying to direct him by holding the back of his head will result in the baby's head not being flexed and will kick in a reflex in which the baby pulls back, just the opposite of what we want when trying to teach him to nurse.

The baby's lower jaw action is critical. Think of the infant as trying to eat a huge club sandwich: place the chin underneath, open wide, close. Help mom to identify when the baby opens wide and when to pull her baby snuggly to her. Having the palm of her hand between the baby's shoulder blades with one hand and her other hand supporting her breast facilitates the timing of this action. Without waiting for a wide-open gape, he nurses on the end of the nipple, causing nipple pain, soreness, and cracking. The first-time nursing mom frequently thinks this looks OK and does not correct it, since the baby seems to be getting some milk.

The baby's mouth doesn't have to surround the entire areola. In many women, the areola is much too large to permit that, but the baby's mouth should cover a substantial amount.

Information and visuals on positioning and many other breastfeeding topics is on the excellent web site BreastFeeding Inc from Jack Newman, M.D., FRCPC, a pediatrician at Children's Hospital in Toronto who has also worked for UNICEF. The videos show babies latching and sucking. Well worth a visit to the site.

Breastfeeding Made Simple from Kathleen Kendall-Tackett and Nancy Mohrbacher is another web site and book to refer to. Look for the podcasts under the multimedia section for more information for mothers.

Babies can be nursed in a number of positions:

Cradle (Madonna, across-the-lap) **hold**. This position is the one that is shown in most pictures.

Remember to start with the nose to the nipple, watch baby open wide, place the lower lip under the nipple, and have the baby come up and onto the breast. A better way to begin is to try a variation, the cross-cradle. It is useful for women to learn this way and then transition into the more traditional cradle hold.

The breast that is being used for the feeding is supported by mom's hand on the same side (e.g., right breast supported by right hand). The opposite arm (in this example, the left) holds the baby across mom's lap.

Football (clutch) **hold**. The baby is held along one arm, with his shoulders cradled in the hand e on the same side. Mom's thumb and forefinger cup his neck and head behind his ears.

Side-lying position. Mom lies comfortably on her side with her legs bent and a small pillow between her knees. A pillow behind her back acts as a wedge so she can tilt back slightly and be supported. Whatever she uses under her head is in place. She takes the baby and a rolled up blanket for his back support, gets up on her elbow and uses both hands to roll baby onto his side, nose-to-nipple When the nipple touches his nose, he will tilt and open and she can hug him on. Then she can gently lower her head to her pillow and pull the rolled receiving blanket behind his back (not his head) for support. Mom can drift off to sleep.

Breastfeeding Made Simple

These positions are illustrated and summarized here, another reminder for new moms to refer to for support.

Using Both Breasts.... Ending the Feed

Mom should alternate which breast she offers to the baby first. One way to remember is to use a hair elastic or easy slip-on bracelet on the wrist of the side on which the baby started, then start with the other side the next time.

The baby should nurse as long as he is actively sucking and swallowing at the first breast. Often a newborn needs some prompting with breast compressions a squeeze and hold to keep the milk flowing and the baby drinking, not just sucking as demonstrated here. Keep him awake for the first fifteen minutes. Then let him finish and detach on his own. A burp or diaper change to try to alert the baby between sides is a good option. Offer the second breast. Because newborns nurse often, both breasts need frequent and complete stimulation.

When the baby is finished, he often falls asleep and off the breast on his own. This satisfied, snuggly baby sleeping in mom's arms is one of the great joys of life. The baby should never just be pulled off the breast. Mom can break the suction by inserting a finger in the corner of his mouth, in between his gums, twist and gently push away from the nipple.

Some babies spit up at the end of a nursing session. Mom should have a clean cloth diaper or towel available to wipe it up. Repeated vomiting, however, especially projectile vomiting, in which the liquid shoots out forcefully, is not normal. The medical provider should be contacted.

Some breastfed babies need a burp; others skip this step. Holding the baby at a 45° angle or on the shoulder often brings up the burp. Burping techniques are discussed in chapter 8.

Frequency and Length of Nursing Sessions

Encourage nursing mothers to breastfeed frequently. A nursing newborn may be hungry every one to three hours around the clock. Because breast milk is digested more easily and quickly than formula, a nursing baby needs to be fed more often than a bottle fed baby. Nursing eight to 12 times every 24 hours is definitely expected.

Some newborns are only mildly interested in sucking during the first day and prefer to sleep. These babies may take a few sucks, nap, and suck a little more. Reassure mom that her baby's eagerness to eat will soon increase. For the first few days of practice, newborns need only the small amounts of concentrated colostrum that nature provides, but for the first few weeks, as the milk supply is developing, the baby should be awakened for a feeding after a maximum of three hours with maybe a four hour stretch from the end of a night feeding (set the clock)

A hungry baby may be making sucking motions and noises, put her hand to her mouth, nuzzle against moms breast, or respond to the rooting reflex. It is not necessary to wait for the baby to cry before feeding her. Keeping the baby in the same room as mom all the time enables her to detect early signs of hunger, which she can satisfy before the baby has to resort to crying to get a meal.

Advise mom to remain flexible. She should be prepared to nurse at any time for the first weeks and to follow the baby's lead. Frequent small feedings stimulate milk production and establish the milk supply more rapidly, stimulate the infant's digestion, limit or prevent breast engorgement (see below under "Coping with difficulties"), reduce the newborn's weight loss in its early days, and help bilirubin levels drop to normal levels, reducing the possibility that the baby will develop jaundice.

In the beginning, feedings can last from 15 to 30 minutes on each breast. Not every feeding will last the same amount of time; just as older children and adults don't eat the same amount of food or sit at the table for the same amount of time at every meal. Feedings will shorten as the baby learns what to do and as his stomach becomes large enough to hold more milk at a time. At each feeding, mom should finish nursing with the first breast, and then offer the second. Effective breastfeeding requires some minutes of sustained suckling.

A normal baby doubles its weight in a couple of months. What the baby does is not intended to inconvenience mom. Newborns are supposed to eat frequently. If they are demanding and erratic, there is a physiologic reason for it.

It is important for doulas to know that if it is suspected that a mom's milk doesn't come in, she should be referred to an IBCLC.

How to Tell if Baby is Getting Enough

One concern nursing women have, and a reason some women hesitate to breastfeed, is that they struggle to understand when the baby is getting enough milk. Here are some guidelines to help her determine that her baby is getting enough breast milk. Weight is one, but not right away. Explain to mom that it is normal for a newborn to lose a small amount of weight after birth. Once a normal feeding routine has been established, a baby should regain birth weight and continue to grow. If a mother suspects that her baby is not getting enough to eat or gaining enough weight, refer her to her lactation consultant or care provider right away. For more information go to Low Milk Supply.

In the early weeks, an infant who is receiving enough breast milk:

- Produces several small loose yellow (not white or pale gray, like clay) bowel movements (stools) a day, increasing one per day for the first week of life then leveling out at 5 - 7 per day. (Ex. one poop on day one, two on day two, three on day three...) For the first few weeks, some babies have a bowel movement after every feeding. After a while, the baby will have fewer stools. A breastfed stool looks like seedy mustard after the first few days of meconium.

- Wets six to eight cloth diapers or five or six disposable diapers a day starting around the third or fourth day of life, with pale yellow (not deep yellow or orange) urine. (Counting stools is more reliable than counting wet diapers.)

- Steadily gains weight after the first week of life, usually four to seven ounces per week. (Five ounces is the average for exclusively breastfed babies)
- Feeds at least eight to twelve times every 24 hours.
- Is alert and active sometimes

If mom had epidural anesthesia for the birth, it may have depressed her baby's signals to suck. Sometimes this may not be noticeable at first but present later, when the nursing pair has gone home. If the baby is very lethargic and uninterested in sucking, mom should contact her IBCLC, and be sure to do a weight check every two or three days. The additional IV fluids moms get with either an epidural or cesarean can cause additional weight on the baby and cause the baby's weight loss to appear more dramatic.

These fluids may also cause moms to have more engorgement, which can interfere with establishing milk supply. Educate moms on how to avoid and prevent engorgement, through frequent nursing, hand expression to soften breasts before feedings or between feedings, not allowing breasts to grow hard and firm. See breast engorgement later in this chapter.

Nutrition Basics for Nursing Moms

The section "Meeting the new mother's nutritional needs" in chapter 4 discusses food choices for the breastfeeding mom, because that advice is important, we summarize it here, with additions.

Let's start with a caveat: Babies all over the world get enough milk from mothers who have a wide range of diets. Milk may be produced even under starvation circumstances. The vast majority of women need not fear that they will have enough milk as long as they follow general dietary recommendations, especially for fluids, get some rest, and relax. In fact frequent nursing is much more important than diet in establishing milk supply.

Frequent small snacks are best for new moms, who must keep themselves nourished but who may be too tired to eat a huge meal. Prepare appealing, nutritious snacks and place them in front of her at appropriate times. Help mom get used to grabbing a nutritious snack before sitting down to nurse.

It may be important is to avoid foods that have caused allergic reactions such as asthma or eczema in the mother, father, or a sibling. Babies with close relatives who have allergies or sensitivities to certain foods are more likely than other newborns to develop allergies as well. In such cases, nutritional counseling would be in order. If mom didn't fill out the section of the prenatal questionnaire on family food allergies, ask before you cook. If there is doubt about any particular food, mom should eat small helpings until she finds out whether they affect the baby five to six hours later. It won't take long to learn which foods, if any, distress the baby and should be avoided for now

Avoiding caffeine after noon is well worth the effort, especially if it means getting more sleep because mom stayed away from stimulants that could keep baby awake.

Nipple and Breast Care

Nursing pads, disposable, reusable or folded handkerchiefs can be inserted in the bra cups between feedings to absorb any milk leakage. If mom prefers to wear no bra at all and feels comfortable that way, fine. An overly tight bra can cause plugged ducts and underwire bras should be used with caution. With her medical provider's permission, mom may take Tylenol as needed for discomfort.

The nursing mother should bathe the nipple and areola with plain water only. The little bumps on the nipple, called Montgomery glands, keep the area clean. Soap, alcohol, and lotions are overly drying to the skin and nipples, making any pain or damage worse. Strong soaps remove protective oils in the skin. Mom may wash the rest of her body with soap as usual.

There is no need to apply creams or oils to the breasts or nipples. If mom feels discomfort and asks what she can do, suggest that she rub a little expressed breast milk into the nipples gently after each feeding and let them air dry. (This is a good preventive measure in any case.) Anhydrous lanolin such as Lansinoh (see the section on sore nipples below), often helps heals sore or cracked nipples.

Special Situations

Nursing after a cesarean section, nursing twins, working while breastfeeding-there are very few breastfeeding problems or situations that hasn't been seen before. When a mom you are serving has one of these circumstances, seek out more information and bring in the experts. A great deal of help is out there.

Sick Mom

Most mothers who become ill can and should continue to nurse their infants. By the time symptoms are obvious, the baby has already been exposed and by continuing to breastfeed, she will pass along to the baby the antibodies that mom's body has started to produce. Help mom gather information about her particular situation and with her medical provider, she can make an informed decision about how to proceed. La Leche League has a wealth of information on mothers nursing during medical situations and conditions.

Note that flu-like symptoms can be a sign of mastitis in mom. Mastitis is breast inflammation and can either be an infection or not. Symptoms include fever, pain, redness on the breast and achiness. This usually comes on suddenly rather than building over days. It is important to keep milk flowing to avoid an abscess, continuing to nurse is the proper protocol. Treatments include heat, rest and, non-steroid anti inflammatory medications or antibiotics. (See the section on Breast inflammation - Mastitis. under Coping with Difficulties)

After a Cesarean Section

Whether a mother's cesarean birth was planned or unexpected, assure her that she can still breastfeed. Finding a comfortable nursing position may be more difficult as long as mom is sore or tender from the surgery. The most suitable position may be lying on her side or back with her knees bent and pillows adjusted to provide support (see "Nursing positions for mom and baby," above). She may also sit in a chair or on the bed. Placing a pillow under her arm eases pressure on the incision. Another choice is the football hold, which reduces pressure on the abdomen. She can check with her medical provider to help her find pain medication to reduce her pain while she is breastfeeding.

The Premature Infant

When a preemie comes home, equipment has kept him alive since minutes after his birth. Mom, possibly after a long and frightening wait, takes the baby home and tries to figure out what to do without the equipment.

A woman who is breastfeeding a premature infant needs continued support from hospital staff, her family, and a breastfeeding counselor. Her baby needs lots of patience and love as he learns to breastfeed. Mom will need plenty of support as she feeds the baby after having only pumped her milk; she may have to do both for a while. The support and guidance of a qualified lactation consultant will be an important referral as a postpartum doula.

Help mom to hold the baby and make sure she understands her medical provider's instructions. Remind mom that breastfeeding her preemie has many advantages. Nursing, for example, may reduce the amount of weight the baby loses. Colostrum is especially important to the premature infant, who may be more susceptible to infection than full-term infants. If the preemie can't suck yet, mom can express breast milk, which can be fed to the baby through a tube, with a dropper, spoon or small cup, (or if more than a few days, - with a bottle)

When an infant must be hospitalized for weeks, maintaining a milk supply requires a steady commitment. The mother must express milk frequently from the start to establish a milk supply. Many hospitals provide these hospital grade electric double breast pumps or they can be rented locally. Insurance often covers the cost. If baby is not drinking at the breast, mom should double pump about 15 minutes, eight times in 24 hours. If her milk becomes abundant she can probably pump as few as five times a day.

As the infant gains weight and strength, feeding at the breast becomes possible. Initially, the infant's weak suck may be frustrating, since it may bring out only a small amount of milk. Holding preemies skin to skin increases the production of breast milk. There must be some kind of sensor that triggers it: closeness, temperature, stimulation, and heartbeat. Both research and mothers of preemies prove it works. And the skin-to-skin triggers the synapses in the brain, helping baby respond naturally.

One excellent resource is *Breastfeeding Your Premature Baby* by Gwen Gotsch, published by La Leche League.

Breastfeeding tips and many other techniques for caring for preemies are discussed in *Kangaroo Care: The Best You Can Do to Help Your Pre Term Infant* by Susan M. Luddington-Hoe and Susan K. Golant. The phrase "kangaroo care" refers to the very frequent skin-to-skin contact between parents and preemies that the authors recommend. This contact helps the parents recognize their important role as they take over from the technology that kept their baby alive in the hospital.

Other reading resources include: *The Womanly Art of Breastfeeding* by Diane Wiessinger, Diana West and

Teresa Pitman and *Preemies - Second Edition: The Essential Guide for Parents of Premature Babies* by Dana Wechsler Linden, Emma Trenti Paroli and Mia Wechsler Doron (Nov 9, 2010).

Twins and More

This is a situation that doulas are often hired for, be prepared! The mother of twins needs both psychological and physical support. She may wish to start breastfeeding each baby individually to bond with that baby and get nursing started. Later, she can coordinate feeding the twins together or separately. Mom may find that breastfeeding both infants at once saves time. Twins don't mind being close together. They're used to it. Nursing two at once also raises prolactin levels and helps to produce more milk.

La Leche League is great for helping mom figure out how to place both infants at the breasts. She can sit up and hold them across her lap or use the football hold. Each infant should be fed on both breasts. A good way to accomplish this is to alternate every 24 hours, which breast the baby gets. He or she can go back to "his breast" of the day as often as he needs to without interfering with his twin's meals.

The mother of twins who are totally breastfed produces a quart to a quart and a half of breast milk per day. She must eat a well-balanced diet and get plenty of rest, which means having plenty of help with childcare and housework.

An excellent volume for moms of twins to have around is *Mothering Multiples: Breastfeeding and Caring for Twins or More! (La Leche League International Book)* by Karen Kerkhoff Gromada (Apr 11, 2007), which covers breastfeeding as well as many other aspects of life with twins.

A Doula Speaks

When Heidi was 28, she became pregnant with fraternal twins. All she wanted throughout the pregnancy was to carry the babies to term, have a natural birth, and nurse them. She had already had six children and had nursed them all. She was a La Leche League member and her sister was a La Leche League leader. So she came from nurturers and I was glad.

In her high-risk pregnancy, she nearly went into early labor, but carried those babies for eight more weeks. The day before she went into labor, her blood pressure shot up really high. The doctor told her to go to the hospital, where she was induced. When she was dilated to about 4 cm, she asked for an epidural.

Suddenly she started seizing. The seizures were brought under control, but a little while later she started seizing again. At that point they gave her general anesthesia and did a c-section. She was unable to see her babies, nurse them, or do anything with them for three days.

I got to her house on day 6 postpartum. The babies were being bottle fed at night. She was trying to nurse but was nervous about being able to produce enough milk.

I tried to get them to nurse. They went right on and started to nurse. I stood over her and kept saying, "That's the perfect latch. You look so beautiful," the stuff I always say: "You're doing great. You've got plenty of milk." I kept doing that.

Every day the babies took less bottle milk and more mother's milk. Less than two weeks postpartum, they were eating only breast milk. This woman is amazing. She nurses those twins simultaneously. She's a saint. I tell her that.

The important thing about nurturing breastfeeding mothers is to constantly reassure them with positive statements. That's what does it. You can see their whole posture changing. You can look at them and say, "Look at that perfect latch. That's exactly how it's supposed to be." I can literally watch their muscles relax, but you have to mean it. I find this very easy. These women doubt themselves so much and just need encouragement. They need someone who is confident enough to come in and say, "This is great. You can do it."

Let postpartum moms talk about their birth. They need to. It may be hard on you if the birth experience was difficult. That's what happened with Heidi and me, but she did it. This woman was seizing in the hospital and really thought she was going to die. She thought, "I'm dying and I'm not going to see my babies. I can't nurse them," and then bam, she was given an anesthetic and passed out. She was telling me that, sobbing.

She was crying, but I was smiling inside because I was watching her work through it and of course she had lived and the babies were fine. She just had to talk it through. I did some research and found out that even during uncomplicated vaginal deliveries, women often feel like they're going to die. The next time I saw Heidi, I told her that having those feelings was normal. I hope this helped her to feel better.

Coping with Difficulties: Call the Lactation Consultant

What is a Lactation Consultant anyway? An International Board Certified Lactation Consultant is a health care professional who is an expert in lactation and breastfeeding care and has been certified by the International Board of Lactation Consultant Examiners. There may be other breastfeeding helpers such as volunteer La Leche League leaders who can assist a mother in support and information.

When a clear problem presents itself, referring mom to a lactation consultant is the right choice. In borderline cases, however, it can be difficult to know what to do. Suppose mom has sore nipples, but the baby seems to be positioned well and you can't think of any reason for the problem. Should you wait a day or two or call a consultant right away? When in doubt, offer the suggestion and let mom decide. Mothers feel great when they get lots of breastfeeding support from several capable sources; in contrast, lack of support has caused many mothers to wean. Effective, early support and guidance is very important. So, if you're not sure, always refer to a lactation consultant. Many moms just want to be reassured by an expert that she is "doing it right."

As with many other aspects of being a doula, you will have to use your judgment. Always err on the side of safety. Here are some basic guidelines:

- If mom is engorged and you can't easily soften the breast and get the baby on it, get help right away.
- If mom is debating calling her doctor, she should call.
- If you are ever in doubt about whether mom needs help, let a professional decide.

Whatever happens, assure mom that it has happened countless times before and with help and commitment can be corrected.

Breast Engorgement

Breast engorgement is a condition in which the breast tissue becomes swollen (engorged). If it is severe, the breast feels very hard and is warm to the touch. Often it is painful.

All newly delivered women should expect some degree of fullness on the second to fourth day after birth, when the body is beginning to produce milk but she can probably prevent engorgement. Frequent nursing is the easiest way to keep the milk flowing and avoid engorgement. Proper positioning helps the transfer of milk to the baby; this in turn boosts milk production.

A hot wet washcloth , squeezed out and placed on the breast for a minute before feeding may be helpful. Some one else can undress the baby. Then mom can gently express milk to soften behind the nipple sufficiently for the baby to latch on more easily

Another successful way to soften the breast tissue, widely used in Africa, Asia, and South America, is to "comb" the breast gently, using a real comb, with a light stroking motion from the outer breast toward the nipple, repeating all around the breast. Yet another method is for mom to gently express some milk by hand or with an electric or manual pump before nursing. The point is to promote milk flow and soften the breast for easier latch-on. The baby will take care of the rest.

Between feedings, a bag of frozen peas placed over the breast can relieve pain or you can ask mom at the beginning of the feeding for permission to make some ice packs using disposable diapers. Soak 2 or 4 diapers (depending on the size of mom's breasts) by running cold water into the diaper from one end to the other. Rock the diaper back and forth to evenly wet it. Hold the diaper vertical to drain out excess water. Put each diaper in the freezer separate and in a U shape. They should be ready in 30 or 45 minutes - very cold but not rock-hard. These diapers can be stored somewhere for the next feeding.

Severe engorgement usually resolves within 48 hours. After the feeding, mom can lay on her back with the ice packs reducing swelling. Reclining helps those extra fluids which is not the milk, drain back into her torso.

With the medical provider's permission, mom may take a non-aspirin pain reliever such as acetaminophen (Tylenol). She may gently massage her breasts from under her arm to down toward her nipple. Using different feeding positions may also help. Kelly Mom offers moms a good overview and suggestions for dealing with engorgement.

Green cabbage leaves are another method to reduce engorgement. Studies are few, but mothers find it helps reduce engorgement. Wash and dry a crisp, raw greenish-white cabbage leaf. Cut out the large vein with scissors or a sharp knife. Wrap the leaf or leaves over the engorged breast, holding them n place with either a nursing bra or a cool towel. (If both breasts are engorged, use two leaves, one on each breast.) If the nipples are sore or cracked and should remain dry, cut a hole in an appropriate place on each leaf to allow air to circulate around the nipple. The leaves wilt in about 15 minutes, when they should be removed or replaced and repeated if needed. Most women have reported significant relief within eight hours.. As soon as the pain recedes, the nursing mom should stop the treatments, which might reduce the milk supply if used for too long at a stretch. Here are more instructions for Cabbage Leaves.

Sore or Cracked Nipples

When nipple soreness occurs, it usually happens during the first few weeks of breastfeeding. The nipples become tender, red and hurt when the baby is feeding. Cracked nipples have cracks or separations of the skin in the nipple or areola. They too may be painful when the infant nurses and eventually bleed.

Proper positioning can usually prevent the nipples from becoming sore. Mom should not apply soap, creams, or lotions to the nipples unless there is a crack, then a soapy wash of the nipple once a day is advised. Experienced moms and doulas know that applying a little expressed colostrum or human milk can do wonders for sore or cracked nipples.

Another option for the nursing mother is a pure lanolin product such as Lansinoh or Medela Tender Care Lanolin Cream. These work wonders on everything from sore or cracked nipples to minor cuts and abrasions . They are sold at many drugstores, online and at major retailers that sell healthy and beauty products or baby items. Sometimes companies have free sampling programs for doulas, ask for samples to give to new mothers.

If these methods don't work and nursing continues to hurt, mom should quickly call in a lactation consultant or her medical provider; she might also find suggestions through La Leche League.

Clogged Ducts

Clogged, or plugged, ducts are milk ducts that are not fully emptied and the gathering of milk in a duct causes a hard lump. One hint is mom's complaint of pain in a specific area of her breast. A clogged milk duct may occur at any time during the breastfeeding relationship. Lumpy breasts are common in breastfeeding women, but rarely a concern.

Clogged milk ducts are prevented by completely emptying the breast at each feeding and avoiding tight bras or clothing that prevent the emptying of the ducts. When clogged ducts occur often, contributing factors may include fatigue, stress, and poor diet. Oversupply issues, moms who make high volumes of milk, are also connected with recurring plugged ducts.

Here is one source for understanding and treating plugged ducts.

Breast Inflammation (Mastitis)

Mastitis is a breast inflammation and may or may not be an infection. Mastitis causes tenderness, swelling, redness, and a burning feeling, usually in just one breast. The condition is often accompanied by fever, extreme fatigue, and muscle aches. The mother typically says that she feels as if she is getting the flu. Mastitis may occur at any time during the course of breastfeeding. One cause is the invasion of bacteria into the breast, possibly through cracked nipples, another cause is the breasts become so full that milk is forced out of the milk cells and into the breast tissue where it is seen as a foreign body triggering the inflammatory response.

Frequent breastfeeding helps to prevent mastitis. Encourage and help the mother make a plan to get adequate rest to help prevent and treat mastitis.

Treatment involves heat, rest, and emptying the breast. If the situation fails to improve within a day or mom develops a fever, she should call her medical provider, who is likely to prescribe an antibiotic. If a mom has mastitis, you may refer her to a lactation consultant for latch difficulties, possible tongue-tie, plugged ducts or possible maternal anemia. Also ask if she's been wearing a tight bra or breast shell, which she should discontinue.

Using a Breast Pump

Doulas often want more information about using breast pumps. We can't go into the techniques in detail here, but they are definitely worthwhile for a doula to know. We suggest that you make an effort to learn about pumping by gathering materials from books, breast pump manufacturers, and the Internet; talking with local La Leche League leaders and lactation consultants; and perhaps visiting a local nursing mom or two, referred by a lactation consultant or La Leche League leader, who are willing to demonstrate their pumping techniques and talk with you about them.

According to La Leche League's The Womanly Art of Breastfeeding, "Preferably, human milk should be refrigerated or chilled right after it is expressed. Acceptable guidelines for storing human milk are as follows. Store milk:

- at room temperature (66-78°F, 19-26°C) for 4 hours (ideal), up to 6 hours (acceptable) (Some sources use 8 hours)
- in a refrigerator (<39°F, <4°C) for 72 hours (ideal), up to 8 days (acceptable if collected in a very clean, careful way)
- in a freezer (-0.4 to -4°F, -18 to -20°C) for 6 months (ideal) up to 12 months (acceptable)"

Read more about Milk Storage.

The Centers for Disease Control and Prevention has similar suggestions.

Two well-known breast pump manufacturers are Ameda and Hygeia The companies provide detailed instructions on how to use their products and many hospitals, birth centers and lactation consultants offer pumps for rent or purchase along with pumping directions. With the Affordable Care Act, breastfeeding pumps may be covered by insurance.

The Breastfeeding Working Mom

Many women want or need to return to work before they stop nursing. An increasing amount of material is available for these moms, and many companies work to offer special nursing/pumping rooms to support nursing mothers. Moms who plan to return to work may start worrying and asking about this almost immediately after the birth. They may even start pumping sooner than necessary.

Be supportive of these women. Advise them that while preparation and planning will be very important, they should relax, get nursing in full swing, and enjoy their babies before they start thinking too much about the day they will leave them for the office. Tell them, "Don't deny yourself the joy of your baby and breastfeeding before you go back to work."

Some women return to work a relatively short time after having a baby, perhaps within weeks. They can gain a great deal by contacting a lactation consultant or La Leche League leader to discuss the details of their personal situations. A good way to help such a mom is to direct her to focus on establishing and enjoying breastfeeding. Later she can make specific decisions that are appropriate for her own situation.

A knowledgeable resource person may have many ideas to share that will help make the transition as smooth as possible. Check books, websites, and other sources of information and support and share these resources with moms.

Reducing stress and time away from the baby is important for the working nursing mom. Help her strategize ways to ease into her return to work. Has she considered returning part time for a few weeks or months? Is this even an option? She might start on a Thursday so that she will only work two days that first difficult week. If she can take Wednesdays as vacation days for a couple of months, she won't be away from her baby for more than two days in a row. If she will be working full time, help brainstorm ways to maximize her time with her baby, how to navigate coming back together at the end of a workday and managing nursing with her schedule.

The baby's caregiver while mom is at work should be supportive of breastfeeding. Otherwise, mom's efforts may be undermined and she may not understand why.

For tips and comprehensive information for working, nursing moms, visit La Leche League International.

When Your Role as a Doula Ends

Become familiar with the breastfeeding support that is available in your community. When you are completing your time as a doula with each mom, make sure she has access to the support she might need, whether in the form of websites, a basic book, membership in La Leche League and information about meetings, or the name and number of a lactation consultant.

By assisting your clients in their first weeks as nursing mothers, you are making an important contribution, not only to their families but also to the future. Thank you, doulas, for your contribution.

Breastfeeding Resources

American Academy of Pediatrics Breastfeeding Initiatives site has a section for professionals and for families.

At Breastfeeding Inc., www.breastfeedinginc.ca At Breastfeeding Inc., our aim is to empower parents by ensuring they receive the most up-to-date information to assist them with their breastfeeding baby. We strive to provide them this information through breastfeeding resources, which include, but are not limited to, free information sheets, video clips, and articles. Some resources, such as books, protocols and videos can also be purchased through the website. The creators of our resources, Dr Jack Newman and lactation consultant Edith Kernerman have collectively seen tens of thousands of babies over the years.

The Breast Crawl: A Scientific Overview Every newborn, when placed on her mother's abdomen, soon after birth, has the ability to find her mother's breast all on her own and to decide when to take the first breastfeed. This is called the 'Breast Crawl'.

Breastfeeding online This takes you to Dr. Jack Neuman's extensive list of articles and handouts such as beginning to breastfeed

KellyMom.com A popular site by a mom and IBCLC with lots of resources for parenting and breastfeeding.

International Lactation Consultants Association. ILCA Use this site to find an International Board Certified Lactation Consultant and to learn more about the organization.

La Leche League International Gives information and encouragement to mothers who want to breastfeed their babies, recognizing the unique importance of one mother helping another to perceive the needs of her child and to learn the best means of fulfilling those needs. You can call for assistance with questions, attend local meetings, become a member and use the extensive website.

MahalaMom.com Check the right hand side of the home page for links to books, videos and a list of links on every imaginable breastfeeding situation.

The Womanly Art of Breastfeeding. Eighth edition by LLLI. Every doula should have a copy of this in her bag to lend to new moms and to use often for information. It is comprehensive information based on years of experience helping mothers breastfeed and utilizing the latest research available.

World Alliance for Breastfeeding Action A global network of individuals and organizations concerned with the protection, promotion, and support of breastfeeding worldwide plus a page of interactive activities for kids under the concerning you.

A newborn baby has only three demands. They are warmth in the arms of its mother, food from her breasts, and security in the knowledge of her presence. Breastfeeding satisfies all three. - *Grantly Dick-Read*

Glossary of terms related to breastfeeding

abscess An infection with pus and swelling. An abscess of the breast is rare and requires prompt medical treatment.

alveoli Tiny milk-producing glands in the breast.

areola The dark, circular area surrounding the nipple.

breast cream A commercial product used to soften breast tissue.

breast massage Gentle stroking of the breast to help milk flow begin.

breast milk jaundice A very rare type of jaundice (see jaundice) that appears between days 4 and 7 after birth. It is caused by an unknown factor in the mother's milk.

breast pad A round, soft, disposable product that is inserted in the nursing bra to protect the clothing of breastfeeding women who tend to leak milk.

breast pump A device used to help a woman express milk from her breasts. Various types include hand pumps, battery-operated pumps, and electric pumps.

breast shells Flexible plastic devices that are worn during pregnancy or between nursing sessions to correct inverted nipples or to protect sore nipples.

clogged milk ducts (see milk ducts, clogged)

collecting sinus, milk sinus The enlarged area in the milk duct system, located beneath the areola.

colostrum A thick, yellowish fluid that can be secreted from the breasts during pregnancy, after delivery, and before mature breast milk begins to flow. Highly concentrated, it contains immunities and antibodies for the newborn.

cue (demand) feeding, feeding on cue A method by which the baby is nursed whenever he gives a hint (cue) that it is time to nurse.

cup feeding An alternative method of feeding newborns who can't nurse yet by placing milk in a tiny cup and letting them drink from it. This method is preferable to switching to bottles if the mother will be able to nurse later. See also finger feeding.

demand feeding (see cue feeding)

duct, plugged Blockage in a milk duct. The usual causes are accumulated milk or cast-off cells.

engorgement Overfull ness of the breast, which becomes hard and swollen.

expression The act of releasing milk from the breast by hand or pumping; also called "milking the

128

breast" and "manual expression. "

feeding on demand (see demand feeding) finger feeding An alternative method of feeding the newborn who can't nurse yet by placing milk on the fingertip and letting him suck from it. This is preferable to switching to bottles if the mother will be able to nurse later. See also cup feeding.

flange The cone-shaped portion of a breast pump, placed against the breast to create suction.

football hold A breastfeeding position in which the baby lies along the mother's side, with his head in front and his feet facing toward her back.

foremilk The thin, watery milk that emerges from the breast at the beginning of a nursing session (see also hindmilk). Foremilk is richer in protein than hindmilk.

hand expression Releasing milk from the breast by hand (see also expression).

hindmilk The milk, high in fat content, that emerges at the end of a feeding (see also foremilk).

jaundice A condition in which bilirubin, a yellowish substance that is a normal part of the blood, accumulates in the bloodstream. This buildup causes the skin and whites of the eyes to acquire a yellow tinge. (The condition is sometimes called "yellow jaundice.") The health care provider should be notified when this condition is suspected. Frequent early nursing (more than eight times every 24 hours) helps to minimize this condition. See also breast milk jaundice.

lactation The production of breast milk.

lactose The type of sugar in breast milk (milk sugar).

letdown reflex Ejection of milk from the breast caused by a physical response by the mother to natural signals, such as her baby's cry or physical stimulation. Multiple letdown reflexes occur throughout a breastfeeding session.

manual expression (see expression)

mastitis A serious infection of the breast that requires treatment by a health care provider. Common causes include a cracked nipple or an untreated plugged milk duct. The mother may have a fever and flulike feeling.

milk ducts, clogged Milk ducts that have not been completely emptied during breastfeeding. The milk that remains forms a hard lump. This condition is also called "caked breasts" or "plugged ducts."

milk sinus (see collecting sinus)

Montgomery glands Small raised areas around the nipple that become enlarged during pregnancy and breastfeeding. The glands secrete a fluid that lubricates and cleans the nipple.

nipple pores The openings at the end of the nipple through which milk is secreted.

nipple shield A plastic or rubber base used to cover the breast as a mother feeds. Nipple shields are rarely and sparingly used because they can reduce breast stimulus and therefore milk production.

nurser system (see supplemental system)

oxytocin The hormone that stimulates the muscles around the alveoli to contract, causing the release of milk. A synthetic form called Syntocinon is sometimes used to induce milk letdown.

plugged duct (see duct, plugged)

prolactin The hormone that stimulates the development of the breasts and the production of milk.

rooting reflex The baby's natural instinct to turn his head toward the side on which his cheek has been touched. Helpful in encouraging the baby to turn toward the desired breast.

supplemental system, nurser system A device that supplies formula to an infant from a narrow tube placed next to the nipple. Supplemental formula is placed in a sterile plastic bag that hangs between the mother's breasts. The extra milk encourages the infant to suck until sufficient natural milk flow can be established.

supply and demand The principle that (when applied to nursing) states that the more a mother breastfeeds, the more milk her body will produce.

weaning Stopping breastfeeding, whether abruptly or gradually.

Night Howls

One line, one alone
In our New Baby Journal:
Our darling, our own,
Is completely nocturnal!

- Maureen Cannon,

Twelve Days of Breastfeeding!

by *Kelliann Mendez* (breastfeeding peer counselor)

On the first day of breastfeeding my mommy gave to me:
colostrum to increase my immunity!
On the second day of breastfeeding my mommy gave to me:
two full breasts and colostrum to increase my immunity!
On the third day of breastfeeding my mommy gave to me:
minimized jaundice, two full breasts and colostrum to increase my immunity!
On the fourth day of breastfeeding my mommy gave to me:
fewer Dr. visits, minimized jaundice, two full breasts and colostrum to increase my immunity!
On the fifth day of breastfeeding my mommy gave to me:
LESS ALLERGIES!... fewer Dr. visits, minimized jaundice, two full
breasts and colostrum to increase my immunity!
On the sixth day of breastfeeding my mommy gave to me:
Zero constipation LESS ALLERGIES!... fewer Dr. visits, minimized
jaundice, two full breasts and colostrum to increase my immunity!
On the seventh day of breastfeeding my mommy gave to me:
teeth and jaw development, zero constipation,
LESS ALLERGIES!... fewer Dr. visits, minimized jaundice, two full breasts
and colostrum to increase my immunity!
On the eighth day of breastfeeding my mommy gave to me:
reduced risk of breast cancer, teeth and jaw development, zero
constipation, LESS ALLERGIES!... fewer Dr. visits, minimized jaundice, too
full breasts and colostrum to increase my immunity!
On the ninth day of breastfeeding my mommy gave to me:
skin to skin comfort, reduced risk of breast cancer, teeth and jaw
development, zero constipation, LESS ALLERGIES!... fewer Dr. visits,
minimized jaundice, two full breasts and colostrum to increase my immunity!
On the tenth day of breastfeeding my mommy gave to me:
decreased chance of diabetes, skin to skin comfort, reduced risk of
breast cancer, teeth and jaw development, zero constipation,
LESS ALLERGIES!... fewer Dr. visits, minimized jaundice, two full breasts
and colostrum to increase my immunity!
On the eleventh day of breastfeeding my mommy gave to me:
bonding and loving, decreased chance of diabetes, skin to skin comfort,
reduced risk of breast cancer, teeth and jaw development, zero constipation,
LESS ALLERGIES!... fewer Dr. visits, minimized jaundice, two full breasts
and colostrum to increase my immunity!
On the twelfth day of breastfeeding my mommy gave to me:
Higher IQ, bonding and loving, decreased chance of diabetes, skin to
skin comfort, reduced risk of breast cancer, teeth and jaw development, zero
constipation, LESS ALLERGIES!...
fewer Dr. visits, minimized jaundice, two full breasts and colostrum to
increase my immunity!

CHAPTER 8

NEWBORN BASICS

Appearance, Behavior, and Care

Mom may ask you whether the baby "looks okay" or is "acting normal." This chapter will give you a general idea of normal newborn appearance and behavior. Doulas can educate parents about reflexes and common conditions such as rashes. Parents love to have this information. With any suspicion that something is not normal, beware of taking even a baby step into medical territory. Advise your client to call her midwife or doctor. Never give medical advice.

Many pediatricians' offices provide regular call hours. A nurse might answer, but the doctor will be consulted, if necessary. Pediatricians expect many calls from new moms and would greatly prefer to hear about issues that are easily resolved than to miss one real problem. New moms are learning what's important, and their providers can help them learn, but only if they are asked.

One of your main goals is to build the family's confidence in caring for their new treasure. Encouraging mom and other family members to do diaper changes as you oversee the process helps them develop nurturing skills. This also has the advantage of providing one more time that you don't have to glove. If mom is sleeping, no one else is around, and you can support her by providing infant care yourself, go ahead, using universal precautions (see chapter 3).

When your client asks you for suggestions about baby care, describe and demonstrate what has been helpful for you and others. Do this humbly; don't act like an authority. You don't want her to feel that you can do things better than she can, especially around issues of carrying, bathing, and caring for the baby. You want to help her feel empowered and confident that she can be a great mom.

Every baby (like every other person) is an individual who likes different things. Encourage mom to discover those likes and dislikes. A nervous mother may try something, find that the baby keeps fussing, and fear she's "not a good mom." Reassure her that everybody (and every baby) has preferences; she just has to learn what her baby likes without the aid of conversation! It is always reassuring for a mom to hear that she knows her baby best, and a doula can point out that even though the baby is only days old, that mom (and dad) has already learned special things about who their baby is and how he/she behaves. Many parents will report to you things like, "He loves when I hold him like this," encourage and reinforce these discoveries.

A Doula Speaks

Sometimes you think you have a simple explanation for something, such as how to put a diaper on, and you'll only have to say it once, but what you think is the simplest thing for someone to understand can really be a challenge for a mom.

I had a client with learning disabilities. She had had tutors during her education. Now she had a baby and there was no such thing as a tutor, and she was extremely insecure about herself and her ability to learn all these things. I guess I was her tutor now.

Every little thing she questioned seven times at least. The way that I communicated had to be very simple. I had to think of even simpler ways of communicating them than usual and repeat them several times because this woman was so unsure of herself.

I did a lot of saying, "What do you think is right? How does this feel? Look at your baby now, doesn't she look happy?" I listened a lot. She told me about growing up.

She had previously had anxiety attacks. So I thought that she could be experiencing a postpartum mood disorder. She asked for many kinds of help from me. Before I stopped working with her, she talked to a psychiatrist. She went on some kind of medication and was better.

How a Newborn Looks

Among a new mother's greatest concerns is whether her baby is normal. This stems from confusion about what a normal newborn looks like. Many people never see a newborn up close until they have one themselves. Media images don't help.

"Newborns" in movies and television commercials are typically much older, even several months old. Visitors who think they're being funny may joke that the baby looks "scrawny" or "like a skinny chicken" or "a shriveled prune" or "a bald old man." Even if they have had babies themselves, they may have forgotten what they looked like in those first foggy weeks, but mothers take almost everything said about their babies to heart, and secretly they may worry, wondering where their idealized baby is.

Remind mom that her baby only recently emerged from her body. Pudgy arms and legs and a fat tummy would have occupied a lot more space in the uterus and had more trouble emerging through the vaginal canal. There's a good reason babies don't fill out for a little while. Soon enough, baby will look round and plump.

Size and weight

During the first few days of life, newborns tend to lose 5% to 15% of their birth weigh, from a few ounces up to a pound, representing fluid loss. As they start to eat, babies regain and add weight rapidly. Therefore, in the first week, moms should not worry if their newborns get a little smaller before they grow larger. This trend should not continue much longer than that, however.

Head

During a vaginal delivery, the baby's head may be compressed as it travels through the birth canal. This can happen safely because the bones in the skull overlap. Unless a facial muscle nerve was damaged during delivery (very rare), the newborn's elongated (molded) head should assume a nice round contour soon.

Assure mom that a newborn's slightly swollen or misshapen head after a headfirst vaginal delivery is common and will round out within a week or two.

Two "soft spots" (fontanels) appear on the baby's head. These permit the head to grow rapidly and do not require special care. The larger spot, toward the front, closes by about age 10 to 20 months. The smaller one, toward the back, closes by the age of six months.

Face

A newborn's face is normally puffy and may have some red splotches, which will gradually fade. Some bruising, which will quickly heal, may have occurred during the journey through the vaginal canal. See also the section on skin, below.

Eyes

The newborn's eyes are dark blue or slate blue. Permanent eye color may not be apparent until six months or more after birth.

Any broken blood vessels in the white of the eye that may have occurred in the trauma of birth will disappear in a few days. Newborns do not usually cry tears, which don't begin until the baby is a few weeks or months old.

Sometimes the newborn's tear ducts are plugged with a slight discharge, which can become crusty. The mother should call the baby's medical provider for advice on how to treat plugged ducts. Using a clean, soft cloth for each eye and gently massaging the lid from the corner of the eye out is often recommended. Many times, breast milk placed in the corner of the eye can clean out any infection and help clear the duct.

Gazing into each other's eyes is an important part of the bonding process for the newborn and her parents. Looking eye to eye while breastfeeding places the baby at a perfect distance for her limited vision. Babies see best at distances of 8 to 12 inches. Babies are very interested in their parents' faces and watch intently.

Doulas should be aware of the importance of eye contact with the baby. Encourage the bottle feeding mother to hold her baby at the same distance as she would if breastfeeding (but without phrasing it that way) to promote the same kind of visual interaction. Parents often talk about their babies' eyes, how alert the baby looks, and how much they seem to be communicating by eye contact.

Newborns can distinguish light from dark and seem to prefer patterns to solid colors. Looking at hanging mobiles or pictures about a foot away from her face helps to stimulate the baby's interest in her surroundings.

Hands and Feet

The baby's hands and feet may have a red or blue tinge for several days after birth even when the rest of the skin color seems normal. The reason is immature circulation, which will correct itself.

Baby's fingernails and toenails can be clipped when they grow too long, but beware that the nails are still connected to the nail bed and clipping too soon may cause some bleeding and can alarm and upset the mom. Often it's not necessary to clip an infant's nails initially, but instead use socks or mittens on their hands to prevent baby scratching himself. Infant nail scissors are available. A time-honored, probably ancient method is for mom to nibble the nails off.

Umbilical Cord

The plastic cord clamp used on the umbilical cord after delivery is removed 24 hours later. The cord will dry up, shrivel to a blackish stump, and fall off by itself in seven to 10 days.

Fold diapers below the cord. Use cotton swabs to cleanse the area at each diaper change. For many years, alcohol was routinely used to help the stump to dry and reduce the chances of infection. Some pediatricians now recommend avoiding the use of alcohol because it can be excessively drying, others still instruct parents to use it. Mom should read the discharge notes from her pediatrician or hospital to learn the current policy.

Instruct the mother to call her pediatrician if she notices a foul odor, discharge, red streaks or bleeding from the baby's navel at any time.

Breasts and Genitals

New mothers may be alarmed to see that the baby's breasts and genitalia are enlarged. The labia may be swollen and separated. Reassure mom that such swelling is normal and gradually subsides. For the first three to five days of life, newborn girls can have a slight discharge from the breasts or a whitish discharge, perhaps tinged with blood, from the vagina. Such discharge is caused by stimulation of the baby's glands by the mother's hormones that were transmitted through the placenta.

The testicles of a newborn boy may be large and swollen. This condition usually goes away, but should be discussed with the provider if mom is concerned. Circumcision, a surgical procedure in which the skin covering the end of the penis (foreskin) is removed, is common but not required for newborn boys. A few medical reasons exist, such as removing the foreskin when it is so tight that it obstructs the flow of urine. In most cases, however, the parents make the decision for personal or religious reasons. Parents should discuss the options with their medical provider before or soon after the birth of a boy. An uncircumcised penis requires no special care in a baby or young child but is cleaned somewhat differently from a circumcised one as he grows older. Special care instructions will be provided for families of boy's with a circumcised penis.

A circumcision is usually performed by a pediatrician or other physician in the hospital within the first few days of life. Jewish families may prefer to hold a circumcision ceremony (bris), with the procedure performed by a professional mohel (pronounced MOY-ull), eight days after birth. Islamic families also have circumcision performed for religious reasons.

Safe, effective medications can be used to reduce pain to the baby during the procedure. A plastic ring is sometimes used instead of a soft bandage. Such rings usually drop off within five to eight days. A small amount of yellow discharge or coating may be seen around the head of the penis for a week. Although full healing takes about a week to 10 days, the site starts to appear healed after only two or three days.

Mom should follow her medical provider's instructions for care. In general, the care instructions at each diaper change are to cover a square of gauze with a glob of petroleum jelly (Vaseline) or A&D ointment, and use the dressing to cover the head of the penis to prevent the diaper or gauze sticking. Mom should call her baby's medical provider if she sees any of these warning signs: persistent bleeding, redness around the tip of the penis that gets worse after three to five days, or the baby's inability to urinate normally within six to eight hours after the circumcision.

Skin

Newborns often have dry skin. Pieces of it may flake off. A high-quality edible oil, such as sesame or olive, may be massaged gently into the baby's skin.

Olive-skinned, Asian, and black babies may have a "Mongolian spot" at the base of the spine, which looks like a large bruise. This normal mark on the skin, a result of extra pigment (melanin), disappears by age 5.

A mild skin rash that fades without treatment is common during the first week of life. The usual places are areas of the body that are rubbed by the baby's clothing, such as the arms, legs, and back. Tiny white spots that resemble pimples (milia) may appear around the nose and cheekbones; these are normal and will disappear on their own. They should not be treated or squeezed.

Advise mom that commercial lotions, powders, and perfumed soaps are more likely to make the rash worse than better, especially if the weather is hot and humid. Plastic diaper covers prevent air from circulating around the buttocks and genitals and may also cause or worsen diaper rashes. The skin inside creases at the wrists and ankles may peel after a few days.

Skin problems that warrant evaluation by a medical provider include a rash that looks like blisters filled with clear fluid or pus, a rash that accompanies a cough or fever, or a rash on a baby who is eating poorly.

Jaundice

Normally, the liver removes bilirubin, a byproduct of the breakdown of the hemoglobin portion of red blood cells, from the bloodstream. In many newborns, especially preemies, the liver hasn't matured fully. Once the liver is mature, it will help rid the blood of bilirubin.

Newborns also lack certain intestinal bacteria that break down bilirubin. Frequent feedings keep the intestinal contents flowing and help to expel excess bilirubin from the body before it can be resorbed into the bloodstream.

Most infants with jaundice don't require any treatment. Your observations and mom's should be reported to the health care provider, who will make that decision. The mother should continue breastfeeding without adding bottles of water. When treatment is needed, the most common form is putting the baby under bilirubin lights ("bililights"). Shining bright light on the newborn causes the bilirubin molecules in the tissues beneath the skin to change chemically in a way that enables the body to get rid of the extra bilirubin without its having to go through the liver first.

If breastfeeding is interrupted because the baby must stay in the hospital for treatment, mom can hand express or pump her breasts to maintain the milk supply. Hospitalization is not always necessary, however. Many home care companies offer equipment for doing light treatments (phototherapy) at home. Suggest that mom ask her pediatrician about this option, which is far more convenient than hospitalization for mother, baby, and family.

Breastfed infants occasionally develop a condition called breastmilk jaundice, in which the level of bilirubin in the blood increases during the first week of life. The cause is not certain but may be because of something in the breastmilk that prevents the excretion of the bilirubin. The condition is not harmful. With breastfeeding jaundice, the reason is likely underfeeding or poor milk transfer, refer mom to a lactation consultant. If the level of bilirubin becomes very high, bililights may be prescribed. All these decisions will be made by the provider, but it's a good idea for you to know the basics so you will understand whats going on.

We don't want to frighten new doulas, but we would like to share a story about a doula who found herself in a difficult position, knew where to seek help, and obtained it. Walking into a family's home, you never know what you will find. Most of the time it will be great, but be prepared for anything. This story also illustrates the value of having a questionnaire for a new client in which the mother fills in her providers contact information as well as having a mother sign a confidentiality form that allows a doula to contact a provider if she deems it necessary.

For more on jaundice in infants

A Doula Speaks

Only once in 13 years have we seen a mother who refused to seek medical attention for her baby even when the doula strongly urged it. The baby's skin was orange, suggesting a high level of bilirubin in the blood (jaundice). The baby was very lethargic, sleeping all the time, not nursing well, and producing too few wet and poopy diapers - a more important sign of trouble than many people realize, and a tipoff to doulas that something is wrong.

The mother rejected the doulas repeated advice to call the doctor. In this case, the signs of jaundice were so clear that we called the pediatrician ourselves, without the mothers permission - the only time we have ever done so. He wanted to see the baby immediately. When the mother refused, the pediatrician called the state Division of Youth and Family Services and had the baby transported to the hospital.

The baby's bilirubin level was 24, high enough to cause permanent brain damage. The baby was treated for 24 hours, after which the mother signed him out of the hospital against medical advice ("A.M.A.").

At this point, the doula felt she could not work with the family any longer and we refunded the money for the remaining hours of doula care. We don't know what happened to the baby or the family. A doula always has the right to leave a family if she feels that she is in danger or if the family's infant care makes her afraid or uncomfortable. In this situation, the doula made a value call, as doulas often must.

The moral of this story is to use your own best judgment in any difficult situation. If you feel that the baby or any other person in the home is in trouble and the family will not seek help on their own, do it yourself. You may feel most comfortable asking the head of your doula service or another doula for her advice before you act.

How a Newborn Functions and Behaves

Newborn babies need feeding and warmth. They need to be dry, loved, and touched, and they need plenty of sleep. Here is a general description of their behavior and the way their tiny bodies work.

Urination and Bowel Movements

The first urine is concentrated. It often contains urates, chemicals that can turn diapers pink. Whether breastfed or bottlefed, a newborn should produce six to eight wet cloth diapers or five or six disposable diapers (which are more absorbent) per day, indicating adequate milk intake. Fewer wet diapers should arouse concern.

The first bowel movement, meconium, is sticky and greenish-black. All newborns should pass meconium within 24 hours of birth. A stool is not considered diarrhea unless it smells bad. A bottlefed baby's stool has a stronger odor and is more solid and darker than a breastfed baby's stool, which is thin, watery, and mustard colored, with a mild smell.

The number of bowel movements per day varies from one baby to another. Some breastfed babies, who tend to pass stools frequently, have bowel movements at almost every nursing session or diaper change. Others can go two or three days with none. Either situation is usually normal. As always, if mom is concerned, she should call her pediatrician or other provider and ask.

Reminder: Always wear gloves when changing a diaper.

Breathing

Newborns' breathing patterns include deep sighs, shudders, and light, rapid breathing as well as gentle, rhythmic breathing. A healthy baby may hiccup, burp, sneeze, and spit up small quantities of milk. Projectile vomiting, which involves so much force that it shoots the liquid across the room, is not normal and warrants an immediate call to the health care provider. If a mother has any concerns about her baby's breathing, she should be encouraged to trust her feelings and contact her pediatrician. RSV is a dangerous infection that affects newborns and young babies, encourage a family to call the doctor if there is any question.

Reflexes

The more you can teach mom and her partner about newborns, cuing them into subtle behavioral signs they might otherwise miss, the more they will appreciate their baby's many qualities and abilities. The point is not to diagnose or assess problems, which is not the doula's role, but to educate parents. Recognizing these cues can help them tune into their baby's reactions.

Here are four of the major normal reflexes in newborns:

- Startle (Moro) reflex. When a newborn hears a loud noise or its position is suddenly changed, the infant may flex its thighs and knees and fan and then clench its fingers, with arms first slowly thrown outward and then brought together as though embracing something. This reflex is often seen when a baby is placed on his back (the position recommended for sleeping babies), swaddling the arms can help prevent a sleeping baby from waking himself with the startle reflex.

- Rooting. When either side of the mouth is touched, the newborn turns its head toward that side.

- Tonic neck reflex (fencing). Turning a newborn's head to one side causes his arm (and sometimes his leg) on the same side of the body to be flung out in the opposite direction.

- Stepping. Holding a newborn (up to six weeks of age) upright and inclining it forward, with the sales of its feet touching a flat surface, can cause the baby to make the movements of walking forward. Show the parents how to try this after a diaper change.

Dr. Marshall Klaus's remarkable, "Amazing Talents of the Newborn: A Video Guide for Healthcare Professionals and Parents" shows ways in which a brand-new baby can react to stimuli and start acting like a real person very early in life. Look for the scenes in the video in which a newborn mimics his grandfather's facial expressions.

Sleep

Newborns sleep as much as 16 hours a day. They don't need absolute quiet to fall asleep, although personality differences in this area emerge early. They enjoy movement and stimulation but will not sleep if overstimulated. For an excessively sleepy baby, especially one who won't eat, a medical provider should be consulted.

A wakeful baby may enjoy being carried about the house in a carrier. New moms must learn to take advantage of both the baby's sleeping and waking times so that she can interact with baby when he is awake and sleep when he sleeps.

At any given moment, a newborn is in one of six states: quiet (deep) sleep, active (light) sleep, drowsiness, quiet alert, active alert, or crying. The quiet alert state is learning time, the best time to talk to the baby and play with him. The video, "Amazing Talents of the Newborn" illustrates this process.

Doulas need to encourage moms to think about all the different options available to help their babies sleep comfortably. Some new moms like to keep a bassinette in the bedroom. Others, especially those who are nursing, like their babies to sleep in bed with them. They often say that sleeping next to their babies gives them a better night's rest. Still others prefer to have the baby sleep down the hall in a crib with a baby monitor. To each her own. Dr. William Sears's book Nighttime Parenting is a recommended resource. A "co-sleeper" is a small, high bed for baby that straps to an adult mattress for togetherness without bed sharing.

Many moms, especially after the early days postpartum, may think there is only one way, the down the hallway, and don't even consider having the baby in bed with them. Yet most of the world sleeps with their babies. During the first year, parenting goes on for 24 hours a day. Sleeping together can be an important part of being close to baby and meeting his needs. Use this resource for safe co-sleeping guidelines.

Couples who felt compelled to set up a special room for baby before the birth often realize once the baby arrives that she is better off close to them in the early days. Baby lived inside mom for nine months, hearing her breathing and heartbeat. It's natural to want to be close to the baby when she is dependent on you for all her needs. Encourage parents to shake off cultural demands and to discover what they instinctively believe is right for them and their baby.

Placing a newborn on his back has proven to help protect against sudden infant death syndrome (SIDS). This topic is included in chapter 3.

A Doula Speaks

Doulas are often the only ones providing guidance to new parents. It is important for us to recognize potential problems with newborns and refer parents to their health care providers. Even as non-medical help, we can sometimes save a life.

Our service was working with a professional family, a first-time mother in her late 30s. The doula arrived for her first day at around noon on a Friday The baby was four days old. The mother told the doula what a "good baby" she had, since he slept all the time and hardly ever wet his diapers. The doula immediately thought, "We need six to eight wet diapers a day for the first few days."

The baby was sound asleep, as usual. After a while the doula asked when the baby had nursed last. Since the last nursing session had been more than four hours earlier, she suggested waking the baby for a feed.

The baby was very lethargic. When he nursed, he vomited with force across the room (projectile vomiting). The mother called this "spitting up." It is not normal. Without alarming the mother, the doula gently suggested that she call her pediatrician to discuss the "spitting up," the low number of wet diapers, and the long time between feedings. The mother said she preferred to wait until her doctors appointment the following Monday.

Still disturbed, the doula called the president of her doula agency. She suggested being more assertive in urging the mother to call her pediatrician. He should at least be notified about the situation and asked whether it would be all right to wait until Mondays office visit before he saw the baby.

This approach worked. The baby was in surgery for a blockage of the esophagus within hours.

We were later told that the baby would probably have died over the weekend had the doula not intervened.

Crying and Colic

Crying is one way an infant communicates. He may cry because he's hungry, lonely, gassy, or irritable, because he feels too hot or too cold, or because it is too loud or too quiet.

Babies do not cry "to exercise their lungs." Crying is not "good for their lungs." All babies cry more during the first four months of life than they ever do again. On the other hand, many babies who are born gently, nursed, and remain with their mothers can have minimal crying. When a mother remains with her baby for the first few days after birth, she learns very quickly to understand all the baby's cues.

Babies provide clues to their needs before they start to cry. Ideally, mom will see baby's movements as he awakes and will hear his smacking sounds as he moves his lips and makes sucking motions. Starting to nurse right away will make it unnecessary for him to enter the distressed mode of crying. A crying baby has a harder time settling down to nurse. The more a mother tunes into all the sounds and actions of her newborn, the easier everything goes. Crying is the baby's final effort to communicate after his subtle clues have failed to bring results.

Parents will learn to understand what their babies are telling them and how to satisfy their needs. They shouldn't let their infants cry for fear that picking them up will "spoil" them. Encourage parents to follow their instincts and soothe their crying babies.

Colic is a word used to describe a condition of extreme fussiness in a newborn even after everything has been tried, a feeding, a clean diaper, no fever or other sign of illness, and so on. The baby cries and cries, perhaps with her knees raised to her chest, and resists all attempts at consolation. Trips and calls to the medical provider reveal nothing. After eliminating the diagnoses of milk intolerance and digestive disorders and checking out the baby for other medical problems, the provider says, "It's probably just colic. Be patient."

The crying tends to be greatest at about six weeks of age, generally long after the doula is gone, but since it may start as early as two weeks after birth, or because you may get another call, it's wise for doulas to know how to help.

Tired moms and dads can be driven to distraction by newborns who wail most of the time. The new parents may feel helpless, inept, useless, guilty, frustrated, confused, anxious, frightened, and weary. They may be convinced the baby is in pain, although that may not be so and hasn't been proved scientifically. They may wonder why they had this unhappy baby in the first place.

If the baby won't be comforted, comfort the parents. Reassure them that no child goes to law school (or kindergarten) with colic; it will go away. Explain that about 20% of infants in the first three months of life cry steadily for several hours a day. Colic affects girls and boys equally and is not related to a family history of allergies. Both breastfed and bottle fed babies can have colic.

This situation has been standard for so many babies for so many years that a number of techniques have been developed in response. They may not work, but often they do, and they are certainly worth trying.

Gas may be the problem. Place the baby on his back on a couch or in the baby bathtub. Gently bend his feet and knees up toward his body. Repeat a number of times. These knee presses help move the gas around and release it. A teensy fart is a good sign!

Colicky and fussy babies like to lie on someone's lap. Placing the baby on his tummy may put a little pressure on his insides, causing gas to come out.

Fussy babies like to lie on something warm, such as a hot water bottle partially filled with warm (not hot) water. The water creates motion and who knows? Maybe it reminds them of that warm, watery place where they lived for so long. In any case, moving a little with the water frequently helps to quiet them.

Another way to provide motion for the fussy baby is to hold him while sitting on a large birth ball. The normal reaction in an adult holding a crying baby is to stand and rock from side to side or to sit in a rocking chair and rock. Walking, pacing, and rocking involve two-dimensional movement. The advantage of the ball is that the parent is resting rather than wearing out the carpet.

Don't fill the ball until it's taut. Leave some "give," so that when you sit on it, it's soft. With your legs, gently rock from left to right at the same time. The result is a gentle bounce up and down. You're expending less energy than when walking but obtaining the same amount of movement. Many babies love a side-to-side and up-and-down rock. At 2 a.m., that's better than walking.

Many parents have reported driving aimlessly for miles in the middle of the night when they found that only the motion of the car could put the baby to sleep. At red lights, some have said, the baby woke up. One substitute for a car might be a swing.

Nursing is an age-old way to calm a baby, but you can't breast feed all day and all night. Parents have also had success with swaddling (wrapping the baby snugly in a receiving blanket or specially made swaddler), talking and singing to the baby, dancing with the baby, letting the baby suck on a pacifier (a controversial issue; you can try your finger, instead), baby massage (see the section on this later in this chapter), and pushing the baby back and forth in a carriage. Showing a baby his reflection in a non-breakable mirror on a baby toy may distract him.

Some babies calm down when they hear "white noise," a constant hum either from a machine designed to provide it or even from a vacuum cleaner. A recording of natural sounds or wind chimes may do as well and be more pleasant for the rest of the family.

Many helpful tips can be found in the book *Parenting The Fussy Baby and the High-Need Child* by Dr. William Sears and Martha Sears.

It's important for the parents of a colicky baby to take breaks. They may choose to alternate four-hour shifts at night so that each one will get at least that amount of sleep in a row. Finding a trusted person to take over once in a while so that the parents can go out for a few hours is crucial for their mental health. Advise parents who are frustrated to always walk away and leave a baby in a safe space instead of holding a baby while a parent is angry or upset. Shaken baby syndrome is real and crosses all economic and cultural lines.

Dr. Harvey Karp's *Happiest Baby on the Block* is another tool for teaching parents ways to soothe a fussy infant. Doulas should read his book, see his movie and understand this method to demonstrate and model for parents another tool for calming their baby.

Hands-On Infant Care

Diaper changes, baths, burping, holding and carrying, these daily tasks soon become second nature to new parents, but for the first couple of weeks, they are learning and figuring things out. Treat new parents with understanding as you help to build their confidence. Point out how great it is to have so many reasons to touch and talk to the baby.

First-time parents have a lot to learn. In the hospital, they are bombarded with information on caring for their newborns, but for at least the first few days after the birth, they are still processing the birth experience. (You can tell because they can't stop talking about it.) They are simply not in learning mode.

By the time they're ready to absorb more information, they're home. Teaching by the medical staff, however excellent, has often failed to take hold. The postpartum doula enters a new mother's life just when she is beginning to have teachable moments again. By understanding that learning curve and not assuming mom remembers what she was taught about baby care, no matter what the hospital staff may have checked off after their teaching sessions, you can make a tremendous difference to your clients. In short, be prepared to start from scratch, but don't insist on it. Watch and listen and then fill in the gaps.

Diapering

Help parents and grandparents find their own way in the diapers they use (for more on diapers, see chapter 2). Before starting the procedure, gather all the supplies you will need:

- Diapers (you may go through more than one in a single diaper change)
- Diaper covers
- Clean washcloth or disposable wipes
- Warm water (if using a cotton washcloth)
- Change of clothes for the baby (you may not know you need it until you get a good look in there)

- Cotton swabs for cord care in the first seven to 10 days after birth
- A&D Ointment or other cream

Show mom how to dampen soft paper towels or wash cloths with warm water. For the first weeks, water is all a baby's bottom needs. There are special "recipes" available online for homemade "Bum Spray" that parents can make on their own if they'd like. Some families will choose to use commercial baby wipes, there are many sensitive types available on the market.

A Doula Speaks

I was helping a first-time mother whose own mother had died. Her father was in her home, enjoying his first grandchild.

The new mom was struggling with breastfeeding and very tired. After one nursing session, mom fell asleep but the baby was still awake. The baby had a bowel movement and needed a diaper change.

I could easily have changed the baby; when mom is asleep, we gladly do baby care, but another family member was present, so why not encourage him to be involved?

So I asked the grandfather, "Would you like to change your granddaughter?" He said, "I've had three children of my own, and I've never changed a diaper. It wasn't something that men did back then." I could have left it at that, but I said, "Even though you've never done it, would you like to learn?"

He said, "Sure." I said, "I'll be right there to help you. let's go and do it together." Because the grandfather was nervous about holding the baby, I carried her to the changing table. I talked him through the job, starting by gathering the necessary supplies. He did everything on his own.

It was one of the most moving diaper changes I've ever seen! The grandfather cried because he was actually caring for his granddaughter.

Changing his first diaper became an emotional experience for him. Grandpa sat in a chair and I brought the baby to him. He rocked his granddaughter to sleep, delighted to have provided an integral parr of her care.

Whether it's for mom or another family member, doulas can facilitate learning in everyone.

Don't do a diaper change yourself unless no one else can. People only grow more nervous after seeing you do it quickly and competently. Give them a chance to mess up and take too long, just as we all did for those first few diapers.

Babies often cry while being changed. This has nothing to do with how "well" the change was done. They may just feel a little frightened at being naked and exposed. This is something to point out to parents.

Keep the room warm. If you wish, play soft music. A music box kept by the changing table or a musical mobile overhead can be pleasant and distracting for both the changer and the changee! If the mother repeatedly listened to a certain kind of music around the house prenatally, the baby will perk up and listen to it.

Bathing

Baby's bath time seems to be one of the most stressful times for new parents. They typically want to be sure the doula is around during that first bath. You can provide instruction, reassurance, and an extra set of hands to pass the towel or soap, but let the family bathe the baby.

Any capable family member who is around should do the bathing. Your role as a doula is to set up the environment and talk the person through it. Family members will enjoy participating, especially if mom is breastfeeding and they may feel that they aren't giving the baby as much one-an-one care as they would like.

The room should be pleasantly warm. Mom may want to play soft music, light scented candles, or use aromatherapy-anything that relaxes her.

The Sponge Bath

During the first seven to 10 days, most medical providers recommend limiting the baby to sponge baths to avoid getting the umbilical cord wet, and even then, to give sponge baths only every two or three days. Mom should get advice on this from her pediatrician.

Some babies like the freedom of nakedness. Others have a stricter comfort zone and prefer to be covered. (Yes, babies can have preferences that specific at such a young age. Stay attuned to the baby's signals and everyone will have a wonderful time.) Keep such babies clothed for most of the sponge bath and wash only one part of the body at a time.

There are many ways to give a bath, remind families that you are showing them one way and that they will find a way that works best for them and that they enjoy. Basics are to wash the baby from cleanest to dirtiest parts and for safety to never ever leave a baby in water alone, not even a tiny bit of water.

You'll need the same supplies as for a diaper change (see above) plus a clean towel. Get everything together. Dip a sterile cotton ball in a basin of warm water. Always start with the face and work down. No soap is necessary on the face.

Gently cleanse each eye, working from the center out. Use each cotton ball only once before discarding it. (A plastic-lined waste basket is handy for this.) Use a clean cotton ball for each eye and facial body part. Then do the nose, mouth, and ears. For the rest of the body, use baby washcloths or cut adult washcloths in quarters. Use one color cloth for washing the face and the rest of the body and a different color to wash the genital area. Refer to this color coding with each bath.

Mom may choose to use only a little mild baby soap for the genital area and none elsewhere on the body. Baby's skin contains its own natural oils. In the first days and weeks, as the body is stabilizing, using water alone may be enough until the body has reached its own balance. If the baby has dry skin, soaps may dry it more.

When the face has been cleaned, wash the neck. Take one arm at a time out of the little shirt. Babies respond best to light pressure. Take this opportunity to massage the arms and hands (see the section on baby massage later in this chapter). Make the experience as pleasant as possible for the baby, as opposed to just doing a quick wipe. As you proceed, pat each body part dry and re-cover it before moving to the next.

Skip the genital area for now and wash the legs and feet. Finally, remove the diaper. Clean the genitals with a color-coded washcloth, using a little mild baby soap and warm water. Dry the area. Apply any healing creams needed. Put on a clean diaper and dress the baby.

Shampoos

Even babies with a lot of hair require shampooing only about once a week. When the baby is dressed and comfortable, hold his head over a basin. Splash water gently and lightly rub a little baby shampoo into his hair. Rinse, then dry well. Another option to avoid getting the fresh clothes wet is to keep the baby undressed during the shampoo or put a towel around the baby and dress him later.

Mom needn't fear washing the soft spots gently. If they are not cleaned, they may start to scale, causing a condition called cradle cap. Mild scales can be removed by gently rubbing a few drops of baby oil into the area half an hour before bathing.

Baths *with* Baby

Once the umbilical cord has fallen off, mom can take the baby into the tub with her unless she has any medical contraindications to this. Babies love to be immersed in warm water with someone they love and to feel (and to remember?) the flow of water around them. The mother's partner may also choose to bathe with the baby for some skin-to-skin time.

There is no absolute time for a bath. Ask mom to consider setting aside half an hour for this special bath at a low point in the day, such as in the late afternoon. She can undress and climb into the tub and then you can pass the baby in to her. No one should step into a slippery bathtub while carrying a baby.

If you aren't around, or after your services in the home have ended, mom can prepare the baby by undressing, taking off all the baby's clothes except a diaper, loosely draping a towel around the baby, and placing him in a baby seat of some kind on the floor next to the tub. Once mom has gotten into the tub and is sitting comfortably, she can reach down, remove the towel and diaper, and lift the baby into the bath. When it's time to come out, she can wrap the baby in a towel, place him back in the carrier, exit the tub and dry herself quickly, put on a robe, and then attend to the baby.

Many families use small plastic baby bathtubs and never think of bathing baby in the family tub. Just make sure the bathtub is clean. If the family has more than one full bathroom, select a tub that is used by the fewest people.

Baths aren't just for cleanliness. The breastfeeding mom can nurse. Parents of colicky babies who relax in warm water may take several joint baths a day to calm them. Some dads have reported crying with joy at their first skin-to-skin contact with their babies. Naturally, the doula will not be around for dad's bath with baby! Mom can help with that one.

Baby bathtubs

Plastic baby bathtubs are usually placed in large sinks or on kitchen counters. The baby is immersed in such a tub more than in a regular bathtub and needn't be covered as much. As with sponge baths, everything should be at hand before the bath starts. The procedure is the same.

Placing a soft towel on the bottom of the tub before adding water helps keep the baby from slipping and helps keep the baby warmer than leaning against the plastic.

Burping

All babies have different burping requirements. Mothers get to know them fast. When a newborn has colic or gas, the parents may need extra time to learn how to burp them. Other babies may hardly ever need burping. Teach parents how to burp the baby.

Popular positions:

- Shoulder burp. Place the baby high up on the burper's shoulder. If the baby needs more encouragement, place his abdomen directly against your shoulder. The pressure of the shoulder massages the baby's abdomen to help the gas come up.

- Using the hand on the same side as the baby-hoisting shoulder, make a "V" with your thumb and forefinger. Hook the thumb under the baby's outside armpit. Rest the forefinger and other fingers against the back of the baby's neck. If baby's head is wobbly, and you held only his back, his head and neck would jerk and fall to the side.

- Hard patting isn't necessary. Rock back and forth or use the other hand to do a gentle back rub.

- Lap burp. Place the baby in a seated position on your lap. Form a "V" with your fingers, as described above, and support the baby's chin with it. Gently rub or pat the baby's back.

- Leg burp. Put baby face down over your thighs, with plenty of room for him to breathe. Rub his back gently.

Holding and Carrying

Encourage parents to hold the baby as much as they want. Remind them that it is not possible to "spoil" a newborn.

Many brands and types of infant carriers are on the market. Sitting in a carrier held against the mother's body stimulates the baby's muscle tone and gross motor activity. He has to move in response to her movements. Beware of baby holders that discourage holding, carrying, and touch, and be aware of recalls, warnings and directions for each and every carrier a family may use. Even if you've used a brand before, re-read directions when you're with another family, some models change and may require inserts or special additions to use with newborns under a certain weight. Encourage parents to read all safety warnings and recommendations.

Carrying babies close is comforting for babies and allows parents the use of their hands. Another advantage is hygiene. If you put a newborn in a stroller or carriage, people won't hesitate to grasp a baby's hand or stick their faces in and coo at the baby, with attendant germs. If mom is holding the baby, people will take a more adult distance and hesitate to press their faces against her chest. If they do, she can feel free to back away.

Baby wearing allows parents to hold their baby close while also being able to get a little something done. In our culture, even with a doula's help, families will need to do things, even minimally, to keep the household running. Wearing a baby allows a parent to chop up a vegetable, take out the garbage or write a thank you note while her baby rests happily. As a doula I often bring my own baby carrier, the Moby wrap with me. With the mother's permission I wear the baby so she can rest and I can keep the household rhythm flowing. Some baby wearing resources: Baby Wearing International and The Baby Wearer.

Putting the baby in a carrier for the first outings may be more comfortable than a carriage for both mom and baby. If you think mom is up to it and has no medical restrictions, you might suggest, "let's put in the baby carrier and take a walk." Help her read the directions for her new carrier and put it on. Fresh air and a little exercise can be emotionally healing while helping mom's muscles to get back in shape all over her body.

The First Outing

Many first-time parents are nervous about taking the baby out for the first time. The usual first outing is to the mother's midwife, obstetrician or other medical provider or to the baby's pediatrician. The doula may be asked to come along.

Follow the doulas rules about transportation: You may accompany a client, but not in your car, and someone else must drive. Public transportation or a taxi are fine, or mom may ask a friend or her partner to drive.

On a visit to the mother's medical provider, hold the baby while mom is being examined to give her a few minutes of privacy. On a visit to the baby's pediatrician, mom may want you to hold the baby throughout the appointment if she has had a difficult recovery, especially from a cesarean section. As always, take your cues from her.

Nutritional Needs of the Newborn

A breastfed baby is getting the perfect food that meets all her nutritional requirements for at least th first six to nine months of life. She will want to nurse frequently, at least eight to 12 times per 24-hour period.

If a new mother is in doubt whether her baby is hungry, she should offer the breast.

At first, meconium will be passed then as her milk comes in, normal breastfed stools look like mustard or cottage cheese and are usually bright yellow in color.

Most bottle fed babies drink 24 to 28 ounces of formula per day in the first six weeks-about 2.5 to 3 ounces every three to four hours. If the baby still seems hungry, the mother can increase the formula by half an ounce at each feeding.

Mothers always worry that their babies aren't getting enough to eat. Reassure them by suggesting that they count the number of wet and soiled diapers produced each day, as discussed earlier in this chapter, and by observing their baby. Is she content after a feeding? Does she doze off to sleep with relaxed, open hands? In general, these are indications of a baby who has had a good feed.

If mom goes out, ask if she wants you to give the infant a bottle (of expressed milk, if she is nursing) while she is gone. If not, and baby frets, head for the rocking chair and polish up those knee-bouncing moves, or use Harvey Karp's 5 S's, to calm the baby until mom returns.

Honoring the Bottle Feeding Mother

We want to honor mothers' choices, including how they decide to feed their babies. Respect and work with your bottle feeding clients. Don't make references to breastfeeding or disparage her choice, but do encourage her to hold the baby during feedings and to use them as special bonding times.

Be tactful in your terminology. Don't mention "breastfeeding." Refer instead to "holding," "closeness," and "bonding." Instruct mom never to prop the bottle and to take feeding times as a special, restful time for her and her baby together.

Infant Massage

Some mothers are hesitant about touching their babies. Infant massage is a well-known and popular way to help parents learn their babies' likes and dislikes regarding touch. It's acceptable to ask mom, partner, or grandparent, "How about taking a few minutes to give the baby a massage?"

Don't do the massage yourself, but do show them how to do it and set up. A session can be as brief as five minutes and still have lasting effects for the both participants.

Learning About and Teaching Infant Massage

Good videos, such as this BabyLove Infant Massage video demonstrate different strokes and tech-

ır, visual way that could never be understood so quickly off the printed page. Seeing an
more effective than reading about it. You can just watch it and replicate it.

t massage have their value, however, and some doulas create lending libraries of books,
movies, and other resources. Others just provide information and let clients purchase these things on
their own. Do what seems most natural to you.

Just as doulas can give moms back rubs like a friend, encourage mothers to do the same for their babies. Explain that you are not a massage therapist, but know the basics and can guide her.

Some mothers need verbal "permission" to touch their babies in this way. With all the reports of sexual abuse, society has become hypersensitive to the negative powers of touch, and many people fear it,
but babies adore and require touch. Studies show that touch is vital and necessary.

Basics of Infant Massage

The room should be comfortably warm. As with any infant-related activity (diapering, bathing, feeding), assemble all the necessary supplies. These include:

- Baby lotion, oil, or cream, to make it easier to slide bare hands along the baby's skin
- A firm surface (can be the floor, bed, etc.) covered with a soft, clean blanket or towel
- A lightweight blanket (especially in cold weather, to keep baby warm)

One good time for a massage is when the baby is a little fussy. A massage may help him calm down or
take a nap. Giving a massage can also be relaxing for mom.

Suggest that mom heed her baby's cues. If he doesn't like to be exposed, she can massage one part
and then cover it as she proceeds. Newborns can make their feelings clear.

Touch should be firm so that it doesn't just tickle. Start with massaging an arm, go down to the hand,
and do a little hand rub. Spend a minute or two on each arm then move on to the back, stomach, legs,
and feet.

The baby will be more receptive at some times than at others. Play it by ear, as with so many aspects
of infant care. It's also good for parents to know that often very young infants don't tolerate massage
sessions for very long, but as they get older and develop a routine, the time baby's enjoy it will length-
en.

Encourage mom to learn more about touching her baby in general. Bath time is wonderful because
you have to touch the baby. She should enjoy herself and not cut bath time short.

For the reluctant or puzzled mom, demonstrate how great it feels. Say, "Let me do it to you. I'll rub a
washcloth down your arm quickly or slowly, squeezing as I go. Would you like to try it with the baby
now?"

Lullaby at 2:00 A.M.

Bottled, bubbled, bedded, clown,
Fast asleep you are. My cup
Runneth over. Almost. Down
You may be. But me, I'm UP!

- Maureen Cannon

Ten Commandments for the Postpartum Mother

By William Sears, M.D.

Dr. Sears is a pediatrician in private practice in Pasadena, California, and a world renowned author and speaker. He and his wife Martha Sears, RN, are accredited La Leche League leaders and the parents of five children.

1 Thou shalt not cook, clean house, do laundry, or entertain.

2 Thou shalt be given a doula.

3 Thou shalt remain clothed in thy nightgown and sit in thy rocking chair as long as thou pleaseth.

4 Thou shalt honor thy partner with an appropriate share of household chores.

5 Thou shalt not give up thy baby to unfamiliar caregivers.

6 Thou shalt take long walks in green pastures, eat good food, and drink enough water.

7 Thou shalt not have strange and unhelpful visitors in thy home.

8 Thou shalt groom thy hair and adorn thy body with attractive robes.

9 Thou shalt not have prophets of bad baby advice in thy company

10 Thou shalt sleep when the baby sleeps.

New Brother

Now is his world tip-tilted. What was womb
And whole-and his-is suddenly awry,
And there are secrets, riddles in the room,
In all the house strange sounds and smells and-why,
She's different too, somehow, she is, his mother.
She hugs him, laughing, calling him "Big Brother,"
And turns away too soon. Why can't she see
How much he doesn't-doesn't!-want to be?

- Maureen Cannon

CHAPTER 9

OFFERING SUPPORT TO PARTNERS AND SIBLINGS

Birth naturally focuses on mothers and newborns, but we must never forget the importance of the partner/co-parent and other children/siblings in the mother's and newborn's life. The doula, on the scene from the baby's first days at home, has a unique opportunity to enlist all family members in infant care and admiration right away. Doulas have the privilege of observing dads and siblings awestruck by their new treasure and learning what it means to be a real parent, brother, or sister as baby settles into his or her first home.

If you wonder whether it's really true that fathers are marginalized in our culture, go to a greeting card store and look at the new-baby cards. How many show a dad?

Fathers

For decades, American dads faded into the woodwork (or their own work), taking a minor role in baby's care. They were excluded from prenatal visits, banned from the delivery room, and elbowed out of the baby's room at home. Fathers understandably took the hint and stayed away emotionally for decades.

For the past several decades, however, dad has been welcomed to prenatal classes and expected to be present at the birth. More than any other generation, dads are participating and involved once the baby comes home, but dad is not always sure what that means, and needs guidance and encouragement, just as new moms do.

Those first days at home with the baby can be crucial in establishing parenting roles. It's all too easy to let mom do everything. Bringing the other parent into the family circle from the start can go far toward helping dad feel that he is wanted, needed, and adept at caring for his child.

Dr. William Sears, pediatrician and father of seven, has written that "fathers are very nurturing when they are encouraged to take part in holding and comforting their newborns. Given the opportunity, fathers touch, look at, talk to, and kiss their newborns as often as mothers do."

Assuming the Role of a Father

Fatherhood has a different meaning for every man who accomplishes it. Just as the doula's goal is to make the transition to parenthood smoother for new mothers, so we must try to help fathers feel comfortable in their new role. Since almost all doulas are women, we cannot act as role models for dad as we can for mom. As a result, our relationships with new fathers are more complex and definitely more cerebral than our relationships with new mothers, but we can still make a difference.

We need to recognize that the father's fears and concerns during the pregnancy seem to expand after the birth. To understand what's going on in the mind of a typical new father, be sensitive to subtle cues. Imagine dads' complicated feelings. Just a sample:

- Joy and pride
- The thrill of being a parent
- Fear of not meeting his increased financial responsibilities
- Helplessness and uncertainty in his new role
- Resentment about assuming child care duties and household chores
- Jealousy about sharing his wife with an intruder in their home
- Anger at his wife's exhaustion and reduced availability to him emotionally, sexually, and in general
- Hostility at the noisy one who keeps them up at night and interrupts every conversation and meal
- Exhaustion from too much excitement and too little sleep
- Sexual deprivation
- Guilt about any negative feelings he has

Many of these may be unconscious. It is not your job to psychoanalyze. Simply be sensitive to dad's needs to communicate (or not) and try to make him feel included.

Finding Dad's Comfort Level

Some fathers retreat or are less actively involved than you or mom might wish. Don't be judgmental. Gently bring the father into the family circle and work with him at whatever level he makes himself available. He may enjoy bathing the baby or taking a bath with the baby (see chapter 8). Infant massage (see chapter 8 again) is a wonderful facilitator of father-infant bonding. Babies in Australian studies who were massaged by their fathers gained more weight, enjoyed a better relationship with their fathers, and greeted their fathers with more eye contact, more smiling, and more vocalizing than babies who were not massaged by their fathers. The fathers who massaged their babies also tended to have better self-esteem than those who didn't.

The first-time dad is often afraid to handle a tiny newborn. He fears that he will accidentally hurt the baby. (Second-time and third-time dads know better.) Men can have some very strange ideas about what's manly. As one writer found out the minute his daughter was born, 'The baby didn't know that I was a man and that we weren't supposed to relate to one another until she could play football."

Reassure the nervous dad and show him how to care for his son or daughter. Advise mom to let dad take care of the baby in his own way, which is likely to differ in some ways from hers and yours. It's OK for the baby to know that she has two parents. Only by providing hands-on baby care without being constantly corrected or criticized will dad gain the confidence he needs to participate fully. Caution mom not to fuss over dad's ways with the baby. Her approval of his skills will payoff big time. If making even the smallest decision, such as what the baby will wear, always falls to mom, dad will have a much harder time feeling comfortable watching the baby by himself.

Actively give the father specific physical tasks to do with the baby and encourage mom to do the same. Ask dad if he would like to change the diaper, and say you will be right there if he needs you. Ask him if he would like you to show him how to give the baby a bath or change her clothes or put on the baby carrier and walk around the house or the block. Dad's often love to learn the Harvey Karp Happiest Baby on the Block soothing skills which can help them feel confident in soothing their baby.

Despite your efforts, maybe dad will make it clear that he does not want to be involved in newborn care, at least while you are around. If that's the case, back off. In some cases, though, you may feel that the reluctant dad is ambivalent and might consider participating more if encouraged to do so. It might be helpful for him to hear you say that your husband (or another new father that you know or have worked for) felt very confused at first and was sure he could never learn to put on a diaper, but quickly became a champ and you'd be glad to help coach him in that direction, too.

The amount of work required to care for a newborn is mind-boggling to almost any new parent, but dads in particular can hardly believe it. The father of two young sons said, "Hardly anyone is cut out for this kind of servitude. The biggest thing about parenting is surrender. You have to surrender to the rhythm of the child. It's like when you break a horse, every new parent has to be broken by their newborn."

Some women who stay at home full time, even on an extended maternity leave, would like the baby's father to be more actively involved in infant care, but have trouble relinquishing control. If mom has quit her job to be a full-time mom, she may view motherhood as her only remaining domain. It may not take long, though, before she resents having to do most of the parenting chores.

However egalitarian the marriage before, men and women tend to develop gender-specific roles once they become parents. Once a woman becomes a mother, she identifies less as a wife and a worker; but when a man becomes a father, parenthood remains secondary to his role as a worker and a husband. That may be just as well, in a way, since somebody has to be devoted to earning that baby's keep, but the woman who returns to work may expect a lot more cooperation at home than she receives. The more realistic a couple's expectations about parenting before the baby arrives, the more likely it is that the marriage will remain strong afterward.

In a letter to The New York Times, a (female) professor of psychology described a study for which she had interviewed dual-earner couples:

"In the study, men who left child care to their wives often ended up feeling marginal to their children's lives. Having learned false lessons from experience with their own fathers, they mistakenly believed that a father's place with his children could never rival a mother's.

"But today's fathers have a choice, and some are choosing to share child care equally with their wives.

When they provide everyday care-feeding, diapering, bathing, comforting, chauffeuring, the bonds they develop with their children are as deep as those we usually associate with mothers."

Sources of Support for Dad

It's human nature for people to seek the advice of their peers. There are excellent books on new fatherhood, written with insight and humor by dads. We recommend the ones listed under "New father" in the suggested reading list near the end of this manual. You may want to keep one or two in your doula bag to lend to clients. A funny book that presents the situation from dad's point of view can break the ice when the parents of a newborn are stressed out.

Like new mothers, new fathers may feel isolated, at least emotionally, and need to vent. Having even one male friend who is a father can serve as an important outlet. Dads may not realize that discussion and support groups exist to allow them to talk with people in the same situation and compare notes. These groups, often available through a local "Y" or hospital, provide a place both to talk and to hear. Assure dad that joining one does not reflect on his joy as a parent. Everyone needs someone to talk to. Finding the time to attend can be difficult, but once a week may work out. Online chat groups may be better than nothing, and they are available 24 hours a day.

Being a Doula for Dad

Always remember that you are there for the fathers, too. Your goal is to help both parents feel relaxed and confident. The positive attitude and sense of comfort and wonder that you foster in each will feed on the other, creating a solid force for high-quality parenting.

Treat dad as a contributing member of the household. Ask how he is adjusting to new sleep (that is, non-sleep) patterns. A day or two after showing him how to change or bathe the baby, ask if he has any questions. He may not be comfortable requesting additional advice because he has already supposedly learned those tasks. Ask what advice he would give to other new fathers.

It may be dad who is paying your fee. He should feel that they have received a good value. While moms value time spent learning and talking, fathers like to see physical evidence of the doula's presence. A good way to satisfy the family is to leave a basket of clean clothes and a simple, healthy meal. Perhaps what the new parents need most, is to have a quiet meal together while you watch the baby. Then you're giving dad a meal and his wife, at least for a little while.

The new father may feel that you are there to take care of his partner, not him. He may feel out of place whenever you are around or delegate infant care duties to you (whether silently or verbally) because that is what he thinks you are there for. Including him in baby care tasks when he is home will help him relax and assume his parental role. Once you leave, mom and dad will have to take over. Explain that you are there as a helper and teacher.

If the new baby has older siblings, make a point of giving the father time to spend with them. You might also occupy an older child for a while so that the father can get to know his newborn. As is so often the case in doula care, knowing what to do and when to do it requires sensitivity, tact, and timing.

The doula may be the only person who sits dad down and explains how much his attentiveness means to his wife right now. Suggest that he do as Dr. Sears suggests: "Improve his serve." Men who are accustomed to being served by their wives should view postpartum as a time to reverse that habit, Dr. Sears wrote eloquently in Mothering magazine: "Serve your wife breakfast in bed. Take a walk with the baby while mother takes a shower and has some time to herself, preferably in the morning or during the notorious 4:00 to 6:00 PM fussy period. Give your wife frequent 'I care' messages .... Take the phone off the hook when mother and baby are sleeping. Guard the gates of your home against well-meaning but intrusive visitors who might upset the delicate harmony within .... If you sense that outside advice is even slightly upsetting, put a stop to it-even if the baby-raising tips come from your mother."

Advise new dads to be hyper-alert to their wives' needs. They shouldn't wait until mom is sacked out on the floor before they realize she needs some TLC and a meal, even if it's takeout. Sometimes all a man needs is a hint. Others wouldn't respond if you clubbed them over the head. Do what you can. You're the doula!

Tips for the New Father

In your own words, at appropriate times, share this advice with dad. He may not hear it from anyone else.

- Get to know your baby. Cuddle and learn to care for your baby. Touch the baby a lot, even when he or she doesn't need a clean diaper.
- Take some time alone with the baby. Get to know each other.
- Find some time alone with your partner with or without the baby.
- Find some time to be with yourself.
- Be as safety conscious as possible.
- Enjoy being a father. Remember that a father who takes care of his baby feels more comfortable with his child and will gain a special closeness with his child.
- Talk to other men about your feelings as a father. You are not alone.

Some great resources for dads:

Father to Be
Dad's Adventure
Boot Camp for New Dads

Gay Couples and Other Partners

Households can be formed in many different ways. Doulas must expect to be exposed to all sorts of family environments. In one case, a doula worked for two women who had ditched their boyfriends and moved in together before giving birth.

It is no longer uncommon for lesbians couples to have babies by means of adoption or artificial insemination. The lesbian mother may be surrounded by a loving family, a supportive community, or an abyss of ignorance and prejudice. Or she may not have a partner. The situation varies as much as for any other mother.

Gay men are also adopting babies and can use the help of a postpartum doula.

If you are asked to be a doula for a gay or lesbian family, ask yourself some tough questions about your own views and assumptions. Accept the job only if you're sure you can welcome the mother-dyad or father-dyad joyously and non-judgmentally. Help the parents to assume their roles as you would for any other parent.

Siblings: Caring for Older Children

How does a child feel when a new baby comes home? That experience has been compared to watching one's husband walk in the door with another woman and say, "She's going to live with us now. You'll have to share me, but I still love you as much as before."

Being shunted off and left out may be a major concern of the sibling. At first, siblings typically feel jealous and angry toward baby, mother, or both. Negative feelings may be directed at the father, too, who in some mysterious way seems to have been involved with the production of this intruder.

The younger the older sibling, the harder it may be for him or her to accept the new addition. Older children may become quiet and withdrawn, while younger children may temporarily revert to outgrown behavior such as tantrums, bed wetting, talking baby talk, and sleeping difficulties. Such behavior is usually abandoned quickly.

The sibling may act hostile, aggressive, stubborn, or competitive. Perhaps the parents have never seen such behavior in their child before and are dismayed, not knowing what to do. To deal with such problems, the parents can consult their pediatrician or other medical provider and read an almost endless list of blogs, websites or child care books.

Although the new brother or sister may have been described as a playmate, newborns won't be ready to play for a long time. The apparent uselessness of a tiny infant can be disappointing to the older sibling, who may have toys and games ready for action when the baby is carried in the door for the first time.

As you work with siblings, try to understand what they're feeling. Ask. You may get an answer. A doula can be a safe confidante, especially if she welcomes such closeness non-judgmentally. Just as you gave mom and dad permission to express their own feelings about the birth and baby honestly, you can do the same for big brother or big sister.

Listen to the meaning behind the words and respond to that. If the child says, "I hate my brother," don't say, "You know you don't mean that." At that moment, she does! Rather than dismissing expressed feelings, acknowledge them and encourage the child to talk about them. You might say, "You are really angry right now. I'll bet you wish you had your mommy back to yourself. Would you like to read a book together and then we'll see if the baby is finished eating?"

Not every big brother or sister hates the new baby. Some barely react to the situation until the new-ness has worn off, perhaps months later. An older sibling who is very young may not even take the newborn seriously. Many parents worry in advance about their older child(ren) and how they will react then are pleasantly relieved that the sibling seems to be doing just wonderfully with the new baby. Remind the parents not to completely let down their guard, to still be mindful of leaving the baby alone in a room with the older sibling, very often, anticipated negative behaviors come out later.

Many siblings assume the baby will eventually leave, like any guest. A cartoon in The New Yorker de-picted a toddler looking up at parents who have just come home from the hospital carrying a new ba-by. The older sibling says, "I hope you didn't throw the box away!"

A Doula Speaks

In one home, the attitude and behavior of a rather strange eight-year-old girl worried me. She obviously hated her newborn brother. I was concerned that she would harm the baby, whom she called "It."

I expressed my concern to the mother, who explained that her daughter was in therapy and on medication for her mental disturbance. Mom didn't seem concerned about any possible disas-ters, so I tried to put those thoughts out of my mind.

I continued to go to the house, but I continued to worry, too. Nothing troublesome happened as long as I was there. I finished my stint as a doula for that family and never found out whether anything happened after I left. I just hope for the best.

Simple Ideas to Ease the Addition of a Baby to the Family

To work well in a family with one or more siblings, you must be sensitive to the entire range of that family's dynamics. Is the mother afraid that she's neglecting her firstborn? Offer to watch the baby so that she and her older child can have a special cuddle and story time. Is the mother so concerned with the older child's feelings that she has hardly been holding the baby to avoid jealousy? Offer to include the toddler in a cooking project, permitting the mother to have quality time with her infant. Play it by ear and take your cues from what is going on around you.

Giving dad time with the older sibling can forge a bond between them that grows stronger than ever. When mom's friends call and ask what they can do, suggest playing a game with the older child or tak-ing her to the park. She will feel special and the parents will get some time to be alone with the baby.

New mothers rarely understand how long it can take for everyone in the family to feel settled and at ease about the arrival of a new baby. Remind your client that even her own body will take several weeks or more to adjust to childbirth and breastfeeding. Advise her to be patient about reinstating family routines and establishing new ones.

If you have more than one child yourself, it may be helpful to share with your client the reactions you observed in one or more siblings when you brought a new baby home. Similar stories about friends' and other clients' children may be just as effective.

Older siblings very rarely harm new babies. Any anger they express is usually directed at their parents. You can be helpful to a new mother whose feelings are hurt when her firstborn rebuffs her. Tell her that such a response is normal in the early days of siblinghood.

In selected circumstances, a mature older sibling may be invited to assist a parent with baby massage. Doing so places the big brother or sister in a caregiving role while providing a means of demonstrating affection for the baby. If massaging efforts are a tad too forceful, the sibling can sing to the baby, fetch items for diapering, or tell the baby a story during his bath.

When thinking about what to say and do to relieve tension related to siblings, let the situation be your guide. You will know instinctively when to be encouraging and when to keep your opinions to yourself. Child rearing is a highly personal issue. Only the parents can set limits for acceptable behavior, whether you agree with their decisions or not. Be sensitive to the fact that the parents may find it difficult themselves to see their older child displaced by an infant in the amount of time and attention they can spare.

Its a good idea to tote in your doula bag several good books to read to newborns' older siblings. Browse in bookstores and catalogs and see what appeals to you. The variety is wide. Ask the librarian in the children's room of your local library for suggestions. Start your own collection of books that you have read to your own children or friends' children or that you happen to like. Choose books that can be read aloud from cover to cover in five to 10 minutes. You won't have a lot of time to spare but will want to give siblings some special time and attention. It's better to finish reading a short book than to stop in the middle of a long one.

Books that cover a wide range of ages are best. One terrific picture book is *The Bad Island* by William Steig. It's simple enough to appeal to preschoolers and sophisticated enough to deliver a message to a child as old as 11 or more. Besides being fun to read, the story presents a wonderful allegory for positive thinking.

A book recommended for ages 4 through 8, but suitable for younger children as well, is the classic *A Baby Sister for Frances* by Russell Hoban with charming illustrations by Lillian Hoban. This timeless tale appeals to all. Frances the badger has a little trouble coping with the infant badger in the house, but comes around. Your client's children will, too.

New Father

And so I have a daughter. I'm
At ease at last with fact and phrase
And you, small girl. How long a time
It took, how many wondering days
Before I-clumsy-could begin
To welcome you, sweet alien,
And mine, my daughter. Tried for size
Upon my tongue, the phrase has its
Own age-old rightness. Ah, how wise
You look. It fits! How well it fits.

- Maureen Cannon

CHAPTER 10

UNEXPECTED OUTCOMES: CARING FOR THE FAMILY AT A TIME OF LOSS

Greeting a newly enlarged and joyous, if tired, family will characterize nearly every job you take on as a doula. In rare cases, however, things may have gone awry. The baby may be ill and not yet able to come home from the hospital. A congenital anomaly such as cleft palate may require surgery now or later or may not be correctable at all.

The baby may have been born dead. Perhaps a twin or triplet didn't survive, or the baby may have been healthy at first, then died in its sleep, in a tragic situation called sudden infant death syndrome (SIDS) or crib death.

Occasionally parents choose to terminate a pregnancy because an ultrasound scan or amniocentesis found a malformation that was "incompatible with life," that is, the baby would have died almost immediately after birth. Genetic or other testing may have identified something that caused the parents to decide to abort.

Even an anomaly that seems small to you may be devastating to the parents who were expecting a perfect baby. If the parents perceive the situation as a loss, it's inappropriate to tell them how lucky they are. Let them talk.

In any such situation, the parents will be dazed. For doulas, too, infant loss is difficult to grasp. A child born dead represents an overturning of the natural order of events. When people lived closer to nature, they understood and accepted the death of animals and people as well as the death of plants. It was all a part of life. Today, technology has taught us that almost any death should be unnecessary. Death reminds us of our vulnerability and mortality. We agonize over what we might have done to prevent it. Most of the time, we could not have done anything. If visiting a home of bereavement troubles you deeply, you may find it helpful to consult other doulas or a health professional to help you work through it.

Whatever you find in the home, you must be prepared to help the parents deal with it if they want you to. You might think a woman who has come home from the hospital without her baby would cancel your services. That is not necessarily the case. If she asks you not to come, and especially if she has a strong support system at home, you may mutually agree to end your connection there. (Whether to refund her payment, and, if so, by how much, remains your decision.) Many doulas have found, however, that their presence and support promote healing, sometimes for themselves as well as for their bereaved clients.

Psychotherapist Kim Kluger-Bell, having studied the subject intensively, concluded in her gripping book *Unspeakable Losses* that the emotional impact of such a loss is determined not by how long the pregnancy lasted or whether the loss was by chance or by choice but by the parent's hopes, dreams, and fantasies about the baby. Therefore, what your client's pregnancy meant to her considering her childhood and adult experiences will influence the depth of her grief when it ended. Those who have formed a minimal bond with the baby are far less distressed than those who already felt a strong attachment to their baby.

Parents dealing with an infant loss or simply the death of their prenatal image of a perfect baby may experience the classic stages of grieving, as outlined by Elizabeth Kubler-Ross in her seminal book *On Death and Dying* denial, anger, bargaining, depression, acceptance. Getting through all those stages can take a long time, and the doula may not be present for them all. Acceptance may be especially difficult and these stages overlap and recur, not occurring in a neat step-by-step way. It's valuable for doulas to understand the basics. Consider reading works by Kubler-Ross and others to give yourself at least a fundamental background in what to expect of families who are grieving.

A Doula Speaks

A doula showed up at a mom's house for her first postnatal visit. The baby girl was the couple's firstborn. During the one-hour prenatal visit, the doula and client had talked about mom's expectations of the doula and how she wanted her to care for the home. They never talked about loss, nor did the prenatal questionnaire mention it. So the doula knew a lot about mom, who was in her early 30s, but not what turned out to be the most significant item in her history.

Upon the doula's arrival, mom handed her the baby and said she wanted to lie down. Fine. When it was time for a feed, the doula took baby to mom, who nursed and promptly handed the baby back. It was clear that she did not want to spend any time with the baby

After a couple of hours of this, the doula realized that something was not right. She decided to make some positive statements to help the mother bond with the baby but when she said how beautiful the baby was, mom said, "No, she's ugly; she has a funny face. She started talking about the baby in a not-good way.

At the end of her first work session there, the doula left, upset. She had observed an obvious problem in bonding. Mom had shared with her that she was distraught in her new role, but why, and what to do about it7

The doula called me, as the president of the doula service. I said, "You never know what's going on underneath it all. Be open, listen, and try to find out why mom can't enjoy her baby." The doula never met the husband, who was at work during the day.

On the second morning, the doula asked mom an open question: " How are you feeling7 Is anything bothering you?" She wasn't prepared for the floodgate that was released. The mother broke into tears and became hysterical. "When I was 17, I lost my mother," she said. "It hurt then, but I miss her more today. I'm so angry that she isn't here to teach me how to take care of the baby and to hold her first grandchild."

For the next three days, the doula sat on the sofa with mother and baby and allowed her to grieve for the loss of her mother for the first time. After several days of letting go, mom started to hold the baby and was able to bond. Once she had expressed her sorrow, she was finally able to release this block. By the end, she was admiring her beautiful little girl. The doula couldn't believe the transformation.

Sometimes all a distressed mom needs is someone to listen. This woman didn't need a therapist, but a nonjudgmental friend to confide in. She wasn't looking for solutions, just an ear.

For the three days that she and her doula drank tea, hugged, and cried, every night that doula needed a doula herself. She went home, called me, and told me everything that happened and how she felt. She needed to process it.

This doula was able to help because her client shared the issue and vented her anger, but what about situations that aren't so obvious7 The doula can't always know why mom is feeling the way she does. We don't know about all the relationships and losses in her life. It's too easy to conclude that she is a bad mother.

Doulas work in an intimate setting. People can hide things from their families and even from their health care providers, but when you're in your own home with someone for hours a day, it all hangs out.

A final thought: A mom's deep sense of loss can be derived from the loss of a father or sibling, who would have been a grandfather or uncle or aunt to the baby if they had lived. Losing a mother is very painful, but it is not the only painful loss that a woman can feel, deeply, when she becomes a mother.

Not Rare, but Still Taboo

One of the most difficult aspects of coping with perinatal death is that our society has no place for it.

Miscarriage, a lay term for the loss of a pregnancy any time before the fetus is viable (able to live on its own outside the uterus), is so common that many health care providers advise women not to broadcast their pregnancies until they have successfully completed the first trimester, when most spontaneous abortions (the clinical term) take place. Many women who have early pregnancy losses never even know they were pregnant. It is generally accepted that about one in five diagnosed pregnancies is lost. In the third trimester, the loss is usually called stillbirth or fetal demise. That of course would be the kind a postpartum doula would be most likely to encounter.

Yet women rarely discuss previous pregnancy losses, perhaps because the topic is too painful, too personal, or socially unacceptable-virtually taboo, like presenting the results of your Pap smear or mammogram at a dinner party. Furthermore, most Americans do not like to be reminded of death in any form.

As a result, many women think they have never known anyone who had a miscarriage. That is extremely unlikely and once they start talking about their own, if they do, people will start to mention their own or friends' or relatives', suddenly seeming to increase the prevalence many times over. They may suddenly find that their own mothers or mothers-in-law miscarried many years before.

Until a pregnancy loss is spoken about, many women feel that what has happened to them is rare. This makes their confusion and isolation even more devastating. Yet nearly one million known cases of spontaneous abortion or stillbirth have been estimated to occur in the United States every year.

Since most women inevitably take tremendous responsibility for the welfare of the fetuses they carry, how much more like a failure does a woman feel who has "lost" a baby. (Note the term's implied carelessness on her part.)

If pregnancy loss and stillbirth are taboo topics for women, they are far less acceptable to men. Unlike the father's friends, family, and coworkers, the doula can apply herself to encourage the outlet of grief and distress. Some men will not open up to a stranger. Others find tremendous relief in the presence of an allied health care worker whose role in his home is to comfort his partner and perhaps himself.

A Doula Speaks

At MotherLove, Inc., the doula service I ran in northern New Jersey, every time a client has had a pregnancy loss or stillbirth, the doula has had one herself, just by chance. In one case I didn't even know about the doula's personal loss until it happened to her client.

One doula had lost a baby a year before joining MotherLove. She told me that she wouldn't be able to cope with any client who had miscarried. I said we would deal with that if it came up, but she wouldn't have to do it if she was uncomfortable with it.

On her first job, everything was going fine. She bonded well with the family and the parents were delighted with the baby.

On the third day, she arrived to a household in chaos. The baby had died during the night of sudden infant death syndrome (SIDS) also called crib death.

What was the doula to do? She called me and I told her we could find someone else to continue with the family if they still wanted the doula support they had paid for, but since she had already bonded with the family, she decided to go back.

The doula later told me that being in that household at that particular time, talking through the loss with her client and crying together, had helped her to heal psychologically more than she had on her own in the previous year. The experience had done more for her own healing than anything she could have imagined.

Why? Possible Causes

Doctors can determine the cause of spontaneous abortions only about half the time. Possible causes include genetic defects, a cervix that is too weak to hold the fetus inside, infections, immunologic disorders (such as lupus erythematosus) in the mother, and hormone imbalances. Unless and until the cause can be identified, the woman may blame herself. She will certainly think back through every moment of her pregnancy, seeking something she did or did not do to cause the loss. Such delving is even more pronounced in women who have given birth to infants with defects.

The chances of having a miscarriage increase with age. Women having babies in their late 30s and beyond are more prone to spontaneous abortion than in the years when motherhood historically began in the teens or early 20s.

The causes of stillbirths, too, can be a mystery approximately half the time. They may be caused, for example, by improper positioning of the placenta, birth defects, and premature separation of the placenta from the wall of the uterus (in Latin, abruptio placentae, "breaking off of the placenta"). Since the fetus obtains oxygen and nutrients from the placenta, it becomes deprived of these things and dies.

Another cause of stillbirth is an umbilical cord that has become knotted or kinked like a twisted garden hose that won't permit water to run through it. An illness in the mother such as an infection, high blood pressure, diabetes, lupus erythematosus, or preeclampsia can render the placenta unable to do its job.

SIDS

More children die of sudden infant death syndrome in the U.S. each year than of cancer, heart disease, pneumonia, cystic fibrosis, AIDS, and muscular dystrophy combined. Most babies who die of SIDS are not sick, malnourished, abused, or neglected. Factors that may increase the risk of SIDS, but do not cause it, include stomach sleeping and exposure to smoke. (Chapter 3 discusses SIDS prevention techniques.)

A number of cases of deaths ascribed at first to SIDS have been found to have been homicide. Knowing this adds to the guilt that parents feel when SIDS strikes. If there are any siblings, they are likely to be very frightened and confused. Families touched by SIDS need professional counseling.

Expectations of and by the Parents

As Kim Kluger-Bell explains in Unspeakable Losses, written after her second pregnancy loss, women and heir partners are expected to "get over" a birth tragedy rather quickly. Some actually do, but for most women, this loss can be greater than that of any other family member. It is unexpected and out of the logical order of things.

One explanation for this disparity is that only the woman has known the lost baby as "real." The same emotions may apply to losses that the doula is unlikely to encounter in a client, such as ectopic pregnancy, failed attempts with fertility drugs and advanced infertility technologies, and abortions performed for medical or other reasons. You never know what a client may have been through before, coloring her reactions now. To everyone else, sometimes including the father, it was "almost" a baby, so why fuss?

While social and religious traditions and rituals surround the death of a child or adult, the death of a fetus or stillborn baby falls into a black hole. The parents are left to fend for themselves. Friends and family do not automatically take off time from work or return from vacations to attend the funeral. To the majority of the world, the death is a non-event. The woman's doctor, who has seen many such deaths, may find the situation fairly routine. Like well-meaning friends, the obstetrician-gynecologist may respond by urging the woman to "try again."

Even when parents are given the opportunity to view a stillborn baby and to arrange for burial, cremation, or a memorial service, parents who have experienced an ectopic pregnancy or a spontaneous or therapeutic abortion, any of which can be devastating, are often treated as though they have had an illness or surgical procedure. Physical wounds are left to heal; psychic wounds are assumed not to exist. With little consolation from others, partly because most people never even know their friends have experienced such a thing, the loss remains secret, private, unmemorialized, and often unresolved.

Thus the mother, and sometimes the father as well, greet the world after such a loss expecting sympathy and sorrow. Instead, what they tend to find are confusion, embarrassment, ignorance, unintentionally hurtful statements, and silence.

Silence is often the best response to those who have experienced a difficult loss. They are so exposed, so raw, so vulnerable to thoughtless, even if well-meant, remarks.

Things not to say to a family grieving a loss:

"It was for the best."
"He/she was never meant to be born."
"God wanted him/her/them."
"He/she is with God."
"He/she is in a better place."
"You still have other healthy children."
You can always have another one."
"If the baby was damaged, it's better off dead."

Would they say these things if an infant or older child had died? Would they say "You can always get another husband" to a recent widow?

Even religious people do not necessarily welcome references to God, heaven, or the Afterlife. Deep sensitivity is required. The person or couple in emotional free fall tend to remember for years (and to quote verbatim) the comments that stung them at their vulnerable time, particularly from people close to them and from health care workers.

What is the best response? Often it is a hug, the simple statement, "I'm so sorry," and a willingness to listen as the mother cries or talks. She may want to unburden herself. She does not want advice unless she asks for it. Cathy Romeo, coauthor of *Ended Beginnings: Healing Childbearing Losses*, speaks in the voice of a mourning mother or father in "Grieving parent: Enter at your own risk," reprinted after the end of this chapter.

Helping the Other Children

Parents caught up in their own grief after a loss may not have the resources to provide the support their other children need. *These topics are discussed in "Caring for the parents of a stillborn or an infant who dies," an essay by two pediatricians that follows this chapter.

Here are some suggestions for parents who want to be there for their families but don't know what to do:

- Listen to what your child is saying. He could be hurting in ways you can't imagine.
- Never deny or minimize your child's feelings.
- Let your child ask questions. They may be hard ones, but respond honestly. It's OK to say you don't know the answer.
- Don't give extensive explanations using medical terminology. That can be frightening. Keep it simple and keep it brief.
- Feel free to share the confusion you feel yourself. You might say, "We don't know why Billy died. We can't always come up with a reason for everything that happens in life. All we know is that it happened and we feel sad."
- If you feel like crying, go ahead. It would be more confusing for a child to wonder why you aren't crying if you feel so bad. Crying together may help both of you.
- Respond to your child's grief. Hold him and comfort him whether he is crying or not.
- Tell your child how much you love him. Even better, show him. Hold him, rock him, sing to him, and spend time with him. Reassure him by your words and especially your deeds that the dead child about whom you are making a fuss was not the only child who is important to you.
- If a child wishes to be included in the memorial service and related events, permit it.
- Consult your family's spiritual adviser, if you have one, about ways to help your child grieve. A loving relative may serve as well.
- Suggest that your child draw a picture, write a story, sing a song, or even do a dance about the baby and what happened. Creative outlets are often very therapeutic for children as well as for adults.
- Be patient with your child and with yourself.

Older children may benefit from attending sibling grief support groups where they can talk about heir feelings openly without being afraid they will hurt their vulnerable parents even more. Find out whether a local hospital, community organization, or mental health agency offers such a group. If so, obtain copies of the brochure and keep a couple in your doula resource files for distribution to clients as needed.

Trying Again

Until mourning for the lost child is complete, "having another one" is considered unwise. Babies can't replace each other. Incomplete or forbidden mourning can leave a parent with a lifelong emptiness that no number of additional children can dispel. Considerations for the pregnant woman who has experienced a previous childbirth loss are offered in Cathy Romeo's "Pregnancy after Childbearing Loss: How to Cope" following this chapter. Studies indicate that women who conceived within 12 months of a stillbirth after 18 weeks gestation or more, had higher levels of depression and anxiety during pregnancy and the postpartum year than women who had waited for at least 12 months before becoming pregnant again.

In *Unspeakable Losses*, Kim Kluger-Bell states, "It is uncomfortable to witness the sorrow of others: it makes us aware of how powerless we are to control so many aspects of our lives, or to help others manage theirs." In deciding to be a doula, you have chosen to embrace all parts of life, including death. You have pledged to aid, support, and care for women after pregnancy, however that pregnancy may have ended.

Learn more at Our Bodies Ourselves - Pregnancy After Infertility or Loss

A Doula Speaks

The needs of clients who have experienced a prior loss may be very different from those of the usual mom. A case in point was a woman who had previously lost a baby to SIDS. She gave birth to a healthy second child, came home from the hospital, and hired a doula from our service.

The mother could not rest or sleep because she was so nervous that this baby, too, would die of SIDS. All she wanted from the doula was to sit and watch the baby so that she could get some sleep. She had literally been staying up all night staring at the baby to make sure she was still breathing.

Wanting to be of more help than that, the doula tried to be creative. She asked if she could put the baby's bassinet in the kitchen and cook while mom napped, but mom wanted none of it. For her, the entire point of having a doula was to be able to sleep knowing that her baby was still alive.

The baby she had lost to SIDS had died in the first couple of weeks of life. For her, as for many people, the point was to get past that hurdle. After two weeks, she started to believe that her baby would be OK. Since what mom wanted was harmless and the baby was not in danger, the head of the doula service advised the doula to do whatever mom wanted. It was another good example of never knowing what to expect when you start working with a new family.

Sharing and Caring

Ordinarily, doulas should keep their birth stories and other personal reminiscences to themselves or mention them only briefly. Infant death, however, makes women feel so despondent and alone that sharing one's own experience (always refocusing quickly on the client's situation), as in the doula tale about the client whose mother had died when she was a teenager, helps clients to believe that you truly understand what the rest of the world apparently does not. For expressions of the needs of a mourning mom or dad as if in their own words, read Cathy Romeo's "Grieving parent: Enter at your own risk," which follows this chapter.

As in any house of mourning, the family may be incapable of performing the simplest daily tasks. Preparing simple meals, tidying the house, doing laundry, running errands, and answering the telephone (perhaps most of all) ease the transition for the grieving parents. Placing a cup of hot tea before the grieving mother may be your most appreciated gesture of the day. If there are other young children in the house, taking them for a walk or playing a game frees the parents to be alone and quiet for a while without worrying that they are neglecting their children.

For moms with postpartum loss or depression, doulas help them find the resources. Families need that support long after you leave. Also, be sure a mom knows that her milk will still come in, offer resources for her to manage this physical reminder of her loss and to minimize it's discomfort. Within your resources, provide information on local breast milk donation sites, being able to give something may be meaningful to a mother. You might also want to find a way to help her get off the baby mailing and email lists. With mom's permission, perhaps you or a family member can to help unsubscribe her from pregnancy sites or baby blogs.

Looking Outward

Many families have found it helpful to hold a memorial service for a baby who has died whether the death occurred before or after birth. They may plant a tree as a marker of the lost young life. A formal farewell ceremony of some kind, perhaps with readings, can be very healing. If your client has not thought of such a thing, you might suggest it.

Parent groups have arisen in many communities for sharing experiences of stillbirth or other losses. Find out what is available in your area and keep brochures and phone numbers available for families who need them. A selection of many such groups appears at the end of this chapter. Local hospitals and religious organizations often compile such lists and will gladly provide them to you and interested parents.

There are many books on fetal and infant loss which may be beneficial to parents at some point, and helpful to doulas and professionals who may support these families. A suggested reading list is provided at the end of this chapter.

Taking the Time to Heal

Give the parents permission to take the time to mourn their dead baby and not to rush to return to their daily occupations of work, house cleaning, or socializing. Even ordinary distractions such as television can be dispensed with. This is a unique time that is appropriately treated in a unique way.

Hug mom, empathize, and listen. Sit with her and look at a picture of her baby. Tell her how beautiful he was. Validate that this was a birth. If mom has kept a lock of the baby's hair, she may wish to put it in a frame or other special place.

You may be asked to help the parents or father pack up the unused baby clothes, take down the crib, and disassemble the baby's room or to do it yourself if they find those tasks too painful. Take a deep breath and do it, knowing you are performing an important service. Don't suggest dismantling the nursery, though. Stripping away all evidence of the baby's existence doesn't necessarily aid healing.

Nourish the family and allow them to be together. You can't fix this problem for them, but you can help them walk through it. Merely your presence in the home interrupts the echoing silence of the baby who is not there.

Loss, Grief, and Mourning Resources

Grief Watch Resources for bereaved family and professional caregivers, also a store to purchase remembrance items, birth announcements, etc

The World Health Organization: Managing Complications in Pregnancy, Emotional and Psychological Support (a guide for caregivers)

Centering Corporation - A Grief Resource Center - books and information

The Grief Recovery Institute - general information about recovery from grief be it for the professional or the grieving individual

Elizabeth Kubler Ross's Web site, the author of On Death and Dying and On Children and Death many resources and tips for those touched by grief and loss

Perinatal Loss

A Place to Remember - for those who have been touched by a crisis in pregnancy or death of a baby

Aiding Mothers and Fathers Experiencing Neonatal Death

March of Dimes Pregnancy and Newborn Loss Resources

March of Dimes Bereavement Kit - free to those who have had a loss

Waiting With Love - For those who choose to continue a pregnancy knowing their baby will die before or shortly after birth or who learn their newborns will die

EriChad Support Group

Hannah's Prayer - Christian support group for loss from conception through early infancy

Bereavement Services Gunderson Lutheran Medical Foundation - resources for parents and health care providers, information, sales of remembrance rings, memory boxes, and caregiver training

Hygeia - a global community for perinatal health, loss, and bereavement

Baby Loss Comfort

Daily Strength Online Stillbirth Support Forum

MEND Mommies Enduring Neonatal Death - a Christian support group

Pregnancy loss and support program National Council of Jewish Women New York Section - a nationwide support group that coordinates telephone counseling and support groups

Remembering our Babies

SHARE Pregnancy and Infant Loss Support - National organization with resources for loss for parents, friends/family, and professionals, free information packet, support groups and chats, and more

WISSP Wisconsin Stillbirth Service Program for any family who has experienced stillbirth

A TIME - A Torah Infertility Medium of Exchange - a group that helps with infertility and loss from a Jewish perspective.

Carrying to Term - a Web site for parents who choose to carry their pregnancies following devastating prenatal diagnosis.

Babies Remembered - materials and resources for grieving families, from the author of Empty Arms

The Stillbirth Alliance

The Death of a Child, the Grief of the Parents: A Lifetime Journey discusses common and individual characteristics of parental grief, parental grief and a sudden infant death syndrome death, fathers' grief, the impact of grief in special parenting situations, thoughts from grieving parents, and coping with loss and moving on.

The Grieving Child: Helping Children Cope When an Infant Dies provides guidance on how to help children cope after the unexpected loss of an infant sibling or other loved one. It provides information about how children of different ages react to death and how parents and other caregivers can help them. Information about family rituals and suggestions on seeking support services is also provided.

The Loss of a Child

The Compassionate Friends - Grief support after the loss of a child

Bereaved Parents of the USA

First Candle

The MISS Foundation Mothers in Sympathy and Support - For parents, professionals, and friends/caregivers

Loss in Multiple Pregnancy/birth

The Center for Loss in Multiple Birth (CLIMB)

Synspectrum, Multiplicity - Loss, prematurity, and special needs in multiple pregnancy with links to other multiple resources.

Grandparent Support

Alliance of Grandparents, A Support in Tragedy International - support for grandparents who have lost a grandchild and information on how to help their children (the parents of the child)

Infertility

The National Infertility Organization

SIDS

The National SIDS/infant death resource center

The American SIDS Institute

Down Syndrome

National Down Syndrome Society- Information about Down Syndrome

For relatives and friends of a baby with Down Syndrome - what to and not to say

Subsequent Pregnancies following a loss

Babies Remembered Sheroke Ilse website - a kind of guru on this issue

Now I Lay Me Down to Sleep Non-profit photography service. They do amazing work and have a beautiful website.

SPALS Subsequent Pregnancy after a Loss Support

Book recommendations:

All of these are on A Place to Remember's site):

Empty Cradle, Broken Heart, Revised Edition: Surviving the Death of Your Baby

A Place to Remember - some religious undertones, but some excellent resources.

Empty Cradle, Broken Heart

Empty Arms

Help, Comfort and Hope after Losing Your Baby in Pregnancy or the First Year

Life Touches Life - a mother's story of stillbirth and healing

When Hello Means Goodbye

Bittersweet Hello Goodbye

Planning a Precious Goodbye

Waiting with Gabriel: A Story of Cherishing a Baby's Brief Life

This Little While

Remembering With Love

An Exact Replica of a Figment of My Imagination: A Memoir, Elizabeth McCracken

Pregnancy After Childbearing Loss: How to Cope By Cathy Romeo

Cathy Romeo, coauthor with Claudia Panuthos of Ended Beginnings, recommends the following coping mechanisms to women who have experienced a spontaneous abortion, stillbirth, or other childbearing loss and are pregnant again. Many of these concepts apply after the pregnancy as well. Reading these suggestions will give you a good idea of only one small part of the aftermath of losing a baby.

1. Accept some anxiety. Don't label yourself paranoid, but see yourself as healthy and sane.

2. Recognize that this is an exceptionally stressful time and do whatever you can to support yourself through it. Ask for help with meals, home, children, and work. You can't be helped unless you express a need.

3. Take excellent care of yourself physically: good nutrition, vitamin and mineral supplements, massage, exercise, relaxation, visualization.

4. Make a list of everything you can think of that nurtures you. Try to grace each day with at least one self-nurturing activity.

4. Express your feelings. Don't wait until you become overwhelmed. Talk, cry, write. Turbulent feelings, mood swings, or fears may cause difficulties with sexual intimacy. Try to share those feelings with your partner.

3. Try not to worry about bonding with the baby during pregnancy. Bonding happens biologically, beyond feelings. When you are ready to attach consciously and emotionally with your baby, you will

7. At some point in the pregnancy, you may choose to write to your unborn child, sharing only what you feel capable of in that moment.

4. Find at least one supportive friend who will ask often how you are doing and accept what you say without making judgments.

9. Find prenatal caregivers who will support your needs. If you need weekly visits for reassurance, perhaps just to hear a fetal heartbeat, try to schedule them.

10. Draw together a birth team who will support your need to feel as safe as possible physically, mentally, emotionally, and spiritually. Above all else, trust your own inner wisdom to know what you need.

Reprinted by permission of the author.

Caring for the Parents of a Stillborn or an Infant Who Dies

By John H. Kennell, M.D., and Marshall H. Klaus, M.D.

Dr. Klaus and Dr. Kennell are pediatricians, researchers, authors, and speakers of worldwide acclaim. Their work in bonding led them to research the importance of touch and support during labor and birth and then to their groundbreaking studies on the effects of doula care. These studies, performed with stringent scientific methods, have roved the long-suspected advantages of doula care in a way that is acceptable to the medical community.

For many families in the United States, rituals for behavior after the death of a close family member that are standard in most ethnic groups of the world have been abandoned or forgotten. That is particularly true for a stillborn or a newborn who died before leaving the hospital. If you find that your client's baby has died, understanding how she is likely to respond will help you ease her through the first painful days.

Adults in acute grief typically feel sensations of physical distress that occur in waves and last for 20 to 10 minutes; tightness in the throat, choking, and shortness of breath; the need to sigh; complaints about feeling weak and exhausted; an empty or lonely feeling; a slight sense of unreality; and a feeling of increased emotional distance from people or downright hostility. The grieving parents often feel anger, guilt, and a loss of warmth in relationships with other people, including friends who are making an effort o help and even their other children.

Between attacks of yearning or distress, the parents are depressed and apathetic. They feel a sense of utility. For a while, they lose the ability to go about their usual tasks. They may have trouble sleeping or eating. They may think of the baby as if it were still alive and idealize its memory. The mother may "forget" what happened and believe she is still pregnant. Distraction and confusion take over.

As a doula, you will see the parents only for the first week or two, when their feelings and responses are likely to be most intense, but grief over a stillbirth, for example, lasts for at least six months and often far longer.

To resolve what is called their mourning reaction, the grieving parents must allow themselves to express their emotions. Helping parents to speak about their grief can significantly aid their mental health and well-being.

Some mothers who have lost their infants have mentioned an almost overpowering urge to grab another baby and touch it or run away with it. If your client says anything like this, reassure her that these feelings are normal as long as she doesn't follow up on them.

If your client expresses what's called pathological grief, she needs immediate help from a skilled medical or mental health professional who has experience with treating this problem. Watch for the telltale signs: overactivity without any apparent sense of loss; furious hostility or the opposite, a dull, wooden manner; or acting in a way that would be dangerous to herself or others.

When a newborn dies in the hospital, all evidence of its existence may be removed with amazing rapidity, and nothing is left to confirm the reality of the death. The parents may not have any privacy or a comforting individual who allows them to express their grief freely. The physician or other health care provider may not arrange for follow-up contacts with the family to see how the mourning process is proceeding. Information about the results of an autopsy is sometimes delivered in a letter.

In many forward-thinking hospitals today, these old habits are changing, but doulas should be prepared to see parents who have not been offered an opportunity to hold their stillborn babies or even see them. Doulas can help families recreate their memories and lost hopes, which can then be mourned, allowing them to go on with their lives. As a doula, you can make a major contribution to the long-term well-being of the parents and family by doing your best to help them be aware that the baby really was born, did live, and is now dead. Unless the parents mourn now, they may develop unresolved grief that can last for a lifetime.

Almost all parents who have lost a baby can recall their distress and anger regarding the actions and words of relatives and friends. Some parents have commented that even if everyone said everything perfectly, they still could not say it in a way that would be really helpful. One thing they always appreciated was the comment that the baby could never be replaced. To the parents, the baby was as unique as any other child.

Prepare the parents for comments from friends and relatives who do not know how to react to the baby's death. Telling the mother that there was really something wrong with her baby, that it never would have been normal and healthy, or worse, that it is "better off dead," reinforces her belief that she has been inadequate and has produced an unsatisfactory baby. She may think of anything unusual during the pregnancy that could have caused the baby to die-even carrying a toddler around. You can make a difference by reassuring worried mothers that normal behavior does not cause a miscarriage or stillbirth.

Mothers in particular tell about their almost overwhelming and unwarranted feelings of guilt in spite of the explanations of relatives, nurses, and physicians that they had no part in causing the death. Both mothers and fathers report going through a period when they kept questioning why this happened to them.

Adapted and condensed, with permission, from "Caring for the parents of a stillborn or an infant who dies." Chapter 7 in Parent-Infant Bonding, 2nd ed., by Marshall H. Klaus and John H. Kennell. St. Louis, C. V Mosby, 982 (out of print).

Communication between the parents

Most boys in the U.S. are still trained to act "like a man" and not to cry or express sorrow. They may develop a pattern of keeping busy to keep their minds on other matters when a death or serious illness occurs. Many fathers take on additional employment and assume extra responsibilities so they are constantly occupied. This often has the effect of interfering with their communication with their partners, who may feel abandoned and shocked about an apparent indifference to their recent loss.

The father may think that keeping busy is the answer to his partner's sadness, too. You might suggest that it would be desirable to arrange to lighten up on commitments and responsibilities, instead, and to spend more time together as they grieve for their baby.

The parents should keep up their rapport and communication while acknowledging and remembering that everyone grieves in their own way and at their own pace. If the father has been sad during the day, he should come home and talk about his sadness rather than hiding it to "protect" his partner. Talking and crying together will help them heal. Each partner needs to know that the other cares deeply about the loss, too.

Don't be afraid of tears; expect a good deal of crying, but every parent's needs are different. Often your most appreciated role will be as a good listener and empathic person.

Children's reaction to death

The mourning reactions of parents are extremely difficult for children to interpret and understand unless the parents communicate their feelings and explain what is happening. Example: "Mommy and Daddy are sad that the baby died. I don't feel like talking or doing the things I usually do right now, but I'll feel better soon. We both love you very much."

The ideas that arise from a sibling's death may be devastating. A child may feel guilty if she has had angry thoughts about the baby. She may have wished the baby would die and believe her mother is quiet because she "knows" this. Older children can be encouraged to put their feelings into words. They may reveal misunderstandings that no one remotely anticipated.

Children have found their mothers not only different in appearance because of the birth but also radically changed in behavior and responsiveness. Even two to four month old infants are drastically disturbed and depressed when their mothers sit in front of them without speaking or any showing facial expression for several minutes or more.

One feature of mourning is that it is self-centered. Nevertheless, with some encouragement a mother can usually find the extra ounce of strength to embrace her living children and give them some explanation of what has happened.

Recommendations for care

Review these major points about caring for parents after a loss.

- Parents' contact with the infant. If a mother loses an infant any time after she has felt fetal movement (quickening), she usually goes through a long period of intense mourning. Today, parents are increasingly allowed or encouraged to see and handle the infant after death. At first one might think that it is good only to remember the baby as a normal, active infant, but seeing the baby provides clear, visual proof that he baby really died. If this did not happen, the parents may have to work through what happened on their own.

- When the baby is stillborn. When a fetus is discovered to be dead before delivery, both parents should be fully informed and the events surrounding labor and delivery explained thoroughly The father and mother should be together during labor and delivery. An atmosphere of understanding and mutual support should be established between the bereaved parents and the medical staff. If that did not happen, they may become a very confused and angry couple. A sense of nonexistence is exaggerated in women who were heavily sedated or anesthetized during birth and deprived of the memories necessary for normal grief. Parents who have held their stillborn infant or dead neonate report the experience as positive and meaningful.

  If they have any inclination to do so, it is helpful if the parents name the baby. This is another way of acknowledging the child's reality and will help later when they think and talk about the child, and sooner if they have a burial or other funeral ceremony. Some parents have expressed anger that stillborn babies are not issued birth certificates.

- Funeral arrangements. If the parents choose to have a funeral, the experience will facilitate the grieving process. A simple funeral with only the immediate family present is best. When parents decide to have their baby cremated, a small private service in their preferred place of worship is often most suitable.

- Avoiding tranquilizers. We strongly encourage that parents not take tranquilizers or other medications to "calm their nerves." Drugs dull the mourning reaction in such a way that it may never fully develop. The parents are left without having fully worked through the experience. Sometimes a sedative may be taken solely at bedtime.

- Group discussions. Discussion groups for mothers whose infants have died are often useful. Many of the mothers in such groups have mentioned their belief that only a mother who has lost a baby can truly appreciate the pain involved. Similar groups are available for parents who have experienced sudden infant death syndrome (SIDS).

- Other children. Surviving children sometimes feel overwhelmed and somehow guilty or responsible for the infant's death. Help them discuss their feelings. Remind the parents to explain that they are crying because they are sad about the loss of the baby, not because they are angry at the other children, and how good it is to have them nearby. Small children should not be expected to cope silently with extremely distressing situations. If a child needs special guidance, the parents might discuss the problems with a child guidance worker.

- Value of listening. Much of your time may be spent listening, often with long periods of silence or crying. It is time well spent.

Grieving Parent: Enter at Your Own Risk

By Cathy Romeo

Please ...

1. Know that I need you. I may not ask for help (I may be much too numb), but I need to know you're there.

2. Know that I do not expect you to make me feel better or to take away my pain. Right now no one can. I need your support, your acceptance of my need to grieve, and your willingness to live with the helplessness you'll fee!'

3. If you haven't called because you cannot handle my grief and your helplessness, say so. I can truly understand that, and I'll feel better than I would if you used excuses that made me think you didn't care.

4. Try to tolerate my anger, if you can. It's not really you or others who anger me; it's that I lost what I loved. I pray you'll forgive my "unreasonable" outbursts. Sometimes they don't make sense even to me.

5. Don't try to stop my tears. My tears may be hard on you, but they are a healthy way for me to re-lease some of my pain. Crying can be healing; please try to sit with me and let me cry.

6. Don't try to cheer me by comparing "worse" losses. Pain is pain, and mine must be acknowledged.

7. Understand if I can't bear to be with your new baby or attend a baby shower or a family celebration. I do wish you joy, and I truly feel gladness for you, but my grief cannot be shelved or suppressed.

8. Don't tell me that what happened must have been "God's will." Hearing that brings me no consolation right now and only adds to the spiritual confusion and isolation I fee!'

9. Don't expect that hearing "She is with God" should be all that matters to me. I may cling to that belief, too, but I still ache to have her here with me, and I ache to know for certain that she is safe.

10. Don't remind me how lucky I am to have other children or that I can try soon to have another. There is not, nor will there be, a replacement for this child. Love cannot be discounted or replaced ... it simply is.

11. Don't say, "It was better this way-better not to have had him longer." I yearn for one more hour with him.

12. Don't say, "I know how you fee!." No one knows that. Please ask instead how I am today. I'll know what you mean, and I'll be grateful for your caring.

12. Offer specific help: a meal, a laundry done, a free hour. I'm too deeply hurt to think very far

ahead. I barely know what I need in this moment, and asking for help, even when you say "What can I do?," is just too hard.

13. Don't tell me to put this behind me, forget, and get on with my life. This IS my life. I need to grieve. I need to be me. And I need not to forget, but to find a way to remember in love and peace.

15. Don't put a timetable on my grief. Will I ever be "over it"? I hope and expect to someday feel better, but a part of me will always be sad. A part of me will ALWAYS miss my child.

16. Hold me; touch me; tell me that you care; bear with me through this uncharted territory that is my grief.

17. Please don't judge me, but accept me in my grief, and I'll always remember the healing love that you offered me.

Reprinted by permission of the author.

CHAPTER 11

NURTURING YOURSELF

By Carlita Reyes

Carlita (Leola) Reyes is a certified drug and alcohol counselor who works with women with HIV disease in Paterson, New Jersey. She is the mother of two, a doula, and a group meditation counselor. Carlita has used her gift of empowering women by providing education and support and teaching them to care for themselves. Carlita's gentle voice and healing ways have supported, nurtured, and encouraged many doulas. [1]

Caring for others is the hallmark of the doula, but the doula who does not also take good care of herself on a regular basis may be unprepared and unable to care for others.

What does "taking care of yourself" mean to you? Good health, good nutrition, good hygiene, and plenty of rest all play a part. So do loving relationships, the constant observation of human nature, perpetual learning, and taking a gentle approach to newborns, their mothers, and their immediate and surrounding families.

Nurturing yourself involves all that and much more. The effective, confident, comfortable doula takes the time and makes the effort to fortify her own body and spirit. Cleansing breaths, quiet times, stretching and relaxation exercises, and meditation will take you far toward remaining calm in the face of difficult and stressful moments you are likely to face from time to time. You must always be ready to greet and handle the unexpected. For this you must be spiritually and emotionally strong.

Start by exploring the suggestions in this chapter that appeal to you most. Consider giving the others a try; you may find they are easier to accomplish and more meaningful than you had expected. Above all, remember that you are a very important person to your clients and to yourself. How can we nurture other women unless we first love and nurture ourselves?

Relaxation Tips

Make time for yourself. Exercise daily. A brisk walk around the block, an aerobics session, a swim, or bicycle riding can alleviate stress and tension. When feeling stressed, take deep, cleansing breaths. You can do this anywhere. Give your best effort and watch it work.

Invest in recordings of tranquil music. This will surely help you relax, especially during your quiet time. Dedicate to yourself at least one Pampering Day per week. How you spend your time is up to you.

Try these time-honored methods:

> Read a good book.
>
> Drive along a scenic route. Walk on the beach.
>
> Take a candlelit bubble bath.
>
> Treat yourself to a full-body massage, manicure, or pedicure. Ask for a gift certificate for your birthday or a holiday.
>
> Experiment with aromatherapy.
>
> Take up a hobby and incorporate it into your quiet time.
>
> Listen to or play music that makes you feel empowered and inspired. Sing inspirational songs with lyrics that nurture your spirit.

Whatever your choice, make sure this day of relaxation and pampering is all for you. If you enjoy being with others or want to include your partner, plan a group activity that includes relaxation techniques or a romantic dinner for two followed by a walk. If you can walk in the woods or mountains or near water, all the better.

Think of a favorite childhood song; hum or whistle it to yourself when you feel down or discouraged. It will help your inner child to become more patient and safe in the outside world. Believe it or not, the inner child handles a lot of grownup stuff when the adult shuts down.

Tell yourself that you love you. Give yourself a big hug for all the little things you do that make you unique and special in your own way.

Pray in whatever way is right for you. Ask for guidance and clear, sound judgment.

Sort out your priorities. Write them on paper to show a clearer picture of what they are. Doing this will allow you to set standards. What do you consider important and unimportant?

Smile more. It looks good and feels great.

Stretch Time: Being good to your body

Doulas do a great deal of bending, lifting, and other physical labor. Stretching prepares your muscles for these activities. Fit in stretch time whenever you can. Use vacuuming the floor as stretch time for your arms and back. Extend your arms as far as you can when pushing the vacuum cleaner away from you and then pull it all the way back toward you. Use both arms, stretching an even amount on each side.

Laundry time can be stretching time, too. When sorting clothes, place the hamper on the floor before you put clothes in the washing machine. Stretch down slowly and lift up each armload. Be sure to bend your knees if the basket is heavy. Use the same concept when reaching for dishes from kitchen cabinets.

Here's a good exercise to stretch your back. Sit up straight in a straight-backed chair, holding your back flat against the back of the chair. Twist slightly at your waist. With one hand, grab the back of the chair. Reverse.

Another exercise will stretch your neck. Sit in a straight-backed chair. Raise your hands straight up above your head and cross them behind your head. With your arms, gently pull your neck forward. You should be able to feel your neck and part of your upper back stretch.

Other good exercises include neck and shoulder rolls. A big birth ball that's so helpful during labor is a terrific aid for stretching.

Meditation

Anyone can learn this important stress reducer. Many doulas find various forms of meditation an excellent way to relax and recover from difficult moments. Keeping a journal, lighting a candle, or reading inspirational quotations while taking a bubble bath can help you learn how to be still and to quiet your mind.

Individual Meditation

Make sure you'll have at least half an hour of privacy. Choose the most appropriate time for your lifestyle. A morning person who hurries off to do her weekday tasks might choose a weekend or a day when those tasks are not before her.

Select a place that is right for you, whether at home, at a park, or on the beach. Play soft, tranquil music to calm your spirit. Find a daily meditation book or, if you prefer, something religious to read. Use a book that you can relate to. It should include a daily subject and affirmations.

If you go outdoors to meditate, find a quiet spot with a focal point such as a cloud, tree, leaf, flower, or running water. Indoors, your focal point may be any pleasing object in the room. Concentrate on your chosen focal point. Breathe slow, deep, cleansing breaths for about 10 minutes.

Allow yourself to enjoy the moment. After you have enjoyed the breathing meditation, read from your book of daily meditations.

Reduce stress at least once a week with a candlelit bubble bath. Use citrus oil for energy or lavender oil for relaxation. In the tub, you can practice meditation by using a bubble as a focal point or by thinking of a rainbow.

Keeping your eyes closed, imagine yourself on top of the rainbow laughing and playing. The rainbow is a magic rainbow and all its colors have special gifts for you. Yellow is the gift of love; you are embraced by it every time you touch it. Purple represents hope: Each time you touch the purple part of the rainbow, hope pours into your heart. You can make the colors stand for anything that you like. After receiving as many gifts as often as you like, you will know when it's time to end your restorative bath. End your quality time with yourself by telling yourself that you love you!

Group meditation

Keep in mind when doing group meditation that not everyone will be at the same level in this activity. If a person can't be still in the same way as the others, that's okay. However, do make it known that meditation should be something you enjoy and can be used to help reduce stress.

Tranquil meditation recordings are useful to start off with. They assist relaxation and prepare the individual or group for visualization. Ocean sounds, waterfalls, and tropical sounds are all excellent for leading into visualization, or if you prefer, use jazz or opera. You may wish to burn a lavender scented candle during meditation.

Sit in a circle. While the recording plays, use a soft voice to guide the group in a breathing exercise, which will help everyone to be of accord. Start with deep cleansing breaths for no less than 10 minutes. Then move the group into visualization.

Ask participants to think of the most peaceful and tranquil place they can imagine with their eyes closed. Doing this will allow their minds to become peaceful and relaxed. Let participants stay there for a few minutes. Ask them to make cheerful or pleasant sounds (laughter, oohs and aahs) to show their enjoyment. Explain that this activity may be awkward at first, but they'll find that it feels good to soak in their comfort zones for a little while.

Upon hearing the cheerful sounds of the group's enjoyment, slowly guide the group mentally back to the room or other place (such as under a tree) where they are physically.

Affirmation exercises can work very well in a group setting. While everyone is still relaxed, the facilitator softly walks around the outside of the circle and whispers affirmations in each person's ear. You will be amazed at the spiritual bond that will develop among group members.

Ask the group for permission to massage each member's shoulders as you whisper her affirmation.

Inspirational readings

There is an extensive selection of inspirational and self-development books, websites and blogs. Choose one or more that have the potential to be meaningful to you. Some may choose the Bible; others, poetry; still others, books written specifically to be used in this manner.

Once you have found the book or books of choice, you will find delight in them. You will begin to notice subtle but noticeable changes in you. That is a positive thing.

Affirmations

Affirmations are statements addressed to yourself that enhance your self-esteem and spiritual growth.

In an affirmation, "I" and "you" are the same person.

Books of affirmations can be purchased or taken out of the library, there are websites dedicated to affirmations, or you may wish to create your own list drawn from multiple sources or write your own. Some may be more helpful at certain times in your life and others more meaningful at other times.

Here are some examples:

> I am worthy to be loved. God loves me just as I am.
> I am beautiful inside and out. I have a beautiful smile.
> I can achieve anything that I put my mind to do. When I am lonely, I know that I am not alone.
> Prayer works for all things.
> I am a child of God.
> Claim your victories.
> Love conquers all things.
> When I am troubled about what I don't have, I find gratitude in the things I do have. If no one told you that they loved you today, I do.
> I have faith in me.
> I will not let fear dictate my actions. Change is good.
> I can achieve my goals with hard work and perseverance. Share your truest self with someone you love.
> Press through your fears.
> Be passionate about your purpose.
> Self-love opens the door to abundant living.
> Painful experiences are life's way of teaching clarity, vision, and faith.
> Self-love is your cornerstone to building a solid foundation.

Many people tend to reject the simplest compliment. If someone says, "You look nice-what a great dress!" they respond by saying, "Oh, this old thing?" If that reaction echoes your own, practice saying "Thank You," instead.

Even after you become open to the idea of giving yourself affirmations, you may find it difficult or impossible to say them out loud at first. Here's a solution: Write them on colorful pieces of paper and post them on your refrigerator, bathroom or dresser mirror, and on the back of your front or back door where you must see them before leaving the house. Do whatever you must to learn to love and take care of you.

Setting Personal Goals

List short-term and long-term personal goals that include nurturing and taking care of yourself. Your lists will offer a clear look at what you want out of life. Start with a list of short-term goals that can be accomplished fairly quickly. Goals should be written down and should be measurable and include a time deadline. Reaching some of your goals will help you develop the faith and courage you will need to establish those that can only be reached over the long term.

Your short-term goals should be realistic and easy to achieve in a short time. If you can't achieve one of your goals in a reasonable time, examine the obstacles that were in your way. Try to think of another way to reach that goal. Set mini-goals to take steps toward the larger goal each day.

Long-term goals can be challenging and demand persistent hard work. Next to each long-term goal, list the steps necessary for you to meet it and everyone who might support you in seeking it. Reward yourself for each step of progress with a gold star, a special meal, a long walk, or whatever will serve as a small medal of honor in your own mind. Choose the same prize for each step you pass so that you will feel an increasing sense of accomplishment as you reward yourself over and over.

Once you have reached a major goal, treat yourself to a full day of pampering. What denotes pampering to you? Get a manicure and a pedicure, a haircut, a full-body massage, flowers sent to you by you, and a new outfit to praise yourself for all your hard work.

Self-Appraisal: How am I Living?

Doulas should want to make sure they are continuing to be caring and nurturing people bringing peace, serenity, and joy not only to their clients but also to their families and, not least of all, themselves. One excellent way to work this into your life is by keeping a journal.

Record incidents and how you reacted to them. Include as many details as possible. After a short time, you may begin to see patterns of behavior. Writing it all down will help you learn how to describe what you are feeling and to give those feelings their proper names.

Questions that pertain to your lifestyle will suggest themselves to you as you write.

Some questions to ask yourself:

What was my mood when I awoke this morning?

Did I think or say something mean about anyone or to anyone today? Did I allow someone to make me angry?

When I got home from work, did I leave my job outside the door? Did I take time out for me when I came home from work?

What was my day like?

Did someone say or do anything to hurt my feelings? If so, did I speak out about it? How many times a week do I sit down to dinner with my family?

Do I say, "Good morning" even when I'm not in a pleasant mood?

Do I feel resentful of anyone?

Am I guilty of anything?

Have I lied today?

Do I speak immediately about something that has upset me or do I wait and allow my anger or distress to build?

Was I kind to someone today?

Keeping a journal makes you aware of areas that need improvement without bashing yourself.

Further Reflections: The God Box

If you believe that you need spiritual or religious guidance in certain areas, you may wish to create a God Box.

Write down everything you consider too difficult for you to deal with on your own, one thought to each small piece of paper. Place these pieces of paper in the God Box. You don't have to do everything by yourself. If you allow other sources of strength to help, you will experience a stronger freedom than ever before. If you do not believe in God, allow the letters to stand for Good Orderly Direction. Doulas must continually do things to keep ourselves centered and grounded in love.

Doulas Speak about Nurturing Themselves

Being a postpartum doula can be really stressful at times. Take half an hour to soak in the bath or sit quietly in the back yard, do something where you have quiet time to regenerate. It can be hard, but make an appointment in your book even if it's just to leave the house and go for a walk in the woods or do something that you enjoy.

You have to learn when you're getting jammed up to be able to say no to a mom even though she feels like she can't do anything without you. Learn to say no in a gentle way and leave the situation without feeling guilty. Being a doula is for family in general. If your family is pulling you the strongest, trust that and don't second-guess yourself. Just as you help the mom to trust herself, learn to trust yourself.

CHAPTER 12

PROFESSIONAL DEVELOPMENT AND BUILDING YOUR BUSINESS

After taking an approved doula training course, you'll decide whether you would rather work as a solo practitioner, in a formal or informal arrangement with other doulas, or as an employee of a community-based or hospital-based doula agency.

Working on Your Own

Most postpartum doulas will venture out on their own, or perhaps jointly with another doula, this model seems to be how the majority of doulas practice, but we will address working for a doula agency or hospital-based program later in the chapter.

Despite the advantages of placing all marketing, scheduling, and financial obligations in an agency's hands, many doulas prefer to work independently, or do not have the option of an agency in their community. They do their own marketing, define their practice on their own terms, and set their own fees. Private doulas typically charge $20 to $50 per hour depending upon their training, experience and the local market going rates. Call around, connect with other doulas, see the range of hourly fees for your area and determine where you will set your price. Sometimes, new doulas who are looking for certification clients, may charge very little in exchange for the client completing paperwork for them, but it is up to you. Your service is worth something, value what you do and what you can offer and set a fair price.

Although all these activities occupy substantial amounts of time beyond working with clients, many doulas believe that spending that time is more than worth the effort. Getting started as an independent doula may take longer than joining an existing group, but most doulas are able to keep themselves busy within six months.

Establishing your Credentials

Before getting started as a practicing doula, you will need to obtain certain documents that you can show to prospective employers or clients. You will have to complete a course in doula training and another in infant/child CPR and first aid. The rest essentially consist of paperwork. You will insert these documents in your doula binder and carry them with you in your doula bag (discussed later in this chapter).

References and Evaluations

Each time you complete work for a new client, give her a simple evaluation form to complete. A sample that you can modify as desired is provided at the end of this chapter. Attach a self-addressed stamped envelope to make it easy for mom to return it. Explain how important it is for you to have feedback so that you can continue to grow and improve as a doula. You may also want to include an area for mom and dads to write about your service and ask them to check a box if it's okay to use their comments as testimonials on your website and in any promotional materials using just a first name, or first name and last initial. Most families are happy to check "Yes."

The form also should request her permission to give her name to future clients as a reference. You will probably find that most moms are glad to praise the service or to share things they wish had been different. Do a good job and prepare for some glowing compliments.

You may consider asking for a note from a health care provider to share with clients as requested. It's important to have an annual physical examination. Before you start, explain to your provider that you will need a dated note on his or her letterhead stating that you are in good health to work with mothers and newborns. Keep a copy with you and file the original at home.

Professional Liability Insurance

People can sue anyone for anything, and they often do. Will anyone sue you? The likelihood is low, but as with any extremely expensive potential disaster, it pays to be covered. With liability insurance, the insurance company will provide an attorney in case of any such problem and will cover your legal fees.

You don't have to have done anything wrong to need a lawyer. Merely being sued requires that you have one. Even nurses who work for hospitals maintain their own coverage at their own expense because individuals can be sued as well as corporations. It behooves the individual to have her own representation that will work hard on her behalf.

Professional liability insurance for postpartum care providers is available from CM&F Group in New York City. It costs under $100 a year and is well worth the peace of mind. Another option for further protecting yourself is to establish your business as an LLC, a Limited Liability Corporation. Speak with a trained tax professional for details and for help in deciding how to set up your business.

Certification from a National Organization

This document demonstrates that you have taken a course on being a doula such as the DONA International postpartum doula workshop for a minimum of three or I prefer four full days of hands-on training for a total of at least 27 hours. Include your doula training program certificate in your doula binder to present to potential clients or employers while you continue to work toward your certification.

DONA International was the first organization to create and offer training and certifications for post-partum doulas. They continue to lead as the largest doula training organization in the world, but other organizations also offer certification pathways. ICEA, Childbirth International, Doula Trainings International, International Center for Traditional Childbearing, Jennie Joseph's COPE Perinatal Outreach Community Education and CAPPA are among the larger groups. In choosing an organization with which to certify, check out how they market for you once you are certified, how experienced are the trainers, how recognized is the program, how thorough and rigorous are the certification requirements, what do they offer for ongoing education. These and other questions will help you choose the program that is right for you.

Such certification would show that you have taken an approved doula training course and met additional advanced criteria. Among the requirements for certification are reading requirements, evaluations from clients, knowing your area resources, and infant/child CPR certification. Certification is required to receive reimbursement from Medicaid and private insurance as we discussed earlier is becoming a reality in more and more parts of the U.S.

Infant/Child CPR and First Aid

Keep a copy of your card demonstrating that you have taken a course in dealing with resuscitating babies and children and the essentials of first aid. It assures your employer and clients that you can handle emergency situations such as giving the Heimlich maneuver safely to a choking two-year-old. We highly recommend taking a combined course in infant/child CPR and first aid, many classes also cover both infant/child and adult CPR all in one course. To learn where these classes are given in your community, call your local hospital, Red Cross office, YMCA or community school. There is usually a nominal fee. Some ambulance corps offer excellent courses at no charge.

Getting to Know Your Community

Women look to their postpartum doulas as resources for referral to other community services. The first time mother and the woman who has had her other babies in different communities may find it difficult to locate all the resources that her community offers to new mothers. Most pregnant women are intensely focused on the upcoming birth. Few take the time to think beyond labor to what they will need in the first weeks, months, and year with a newborn.

A Doula Speaks

In the childbirth education classes that I teach, I often joke that couples hang on to my every word about labor and birth until they get to the class I do on newborns. At that point, most of the information goes in one ear and out the other. Their focus simply isn't there yet.

When the new parents return for a reunion after their babies are born, I can't believe how little they heard during that class, but they all agree after the fact that we should spend one night on labor and birth, since that will happen in any case and usually in under 24 hours, and the next nine classes on parenting, since that task will consume the rest of their lives.

Before you start as a doula, learn what your community has to offer to new families. This community involvement will serve two purposes. First, you will gather important information to share with your clients. Second, as you educate yourself, you will introduce yourself and the role of a doula to many people.

How to do this? Start with an internet search, find local baby guides and directories, and local parenting publications and read the ads. Talk to childbirth educators and network with anyone remotely related to birth, pregnant mamas, and young families. Local baby stores, photographers, massage therapists, chiropractors, acupuncturists, diaper services, baby furniture stores, exercise classes at a "Y" or gym, breast pump rental outlets, and other such practitioners will be good resources to have in your network.

You are not just talking about yourself and asking for the names of potential clients. You are also letting your contacts tell you about themselves and their services and saying that you will refer your clients to them. Most providers, companies, stores and childbirth educators love to develop professional relationships that are two-way streets. Show genuine interest in them and you will find that your enthusiasm is reciprocated. Distribute copies of your brochure and business cards (more on this later).

Referrals

Once you have gathered business cards, brochures and pamphlets from individuals and agencies in your community and those nearby, you will be ready to make appropriate referrals when needed. Always ask your client to tell the person she calls that you suggested she call and provided the reference's name and phone number. Whenever you receive a call or email ask, "How did you hear about me?" Track your referrals so you can send thank you notes and provide more brochures when their stock seems to be running low. Consider sending holiday cards to thank them for their help. Mother's Day cards are appropriate for many contacts in our business.

Besides the individuals, groups and stores suggested above, here are some additional ones to keep in mind. You may find more in your community.

- Hospitals and birth centers
- Midwives
- Childbirth educators
- Obstetricians
- Pediatricians
- Nurse practitioners
- Instructors in prenatal exercise classes or yoga
- Local chapter of La Leche League
- Maternity clothing stores
- • Holistic health caregivers: chiropractors, acupuncturist, nutritionists, cranial sacral therapist, massage therapists
- Baby furniture stores

- Lactation consultants
- • New Mother's circles
- Instructors in postpartum or prenatal exercise classes
- People who run infant loss support groups
- People who run postpartum depression support groups
- Mother-and-baby or father-and-baby classes, sometimes offered at the "Y"
- Psychologists who specialize in women's issues, birth trauma, postpartum adjustment and relationship changes after a baby is born

Setting Yourself up in Business

Doulas have traditionally been warm, loving people who did not know or wish to know how to put themselves forward as businesspeople. This was once true of nurses, too, but many now run their own businesses and have learned to market themselves. As a result. they have raised their professional image as well as their income. If you work alone, you must learn many simple business practices to build your business and keep viable.

One program I highly recommend is Marie Forleo's —B-School. It is only offered once a year. I always share on my weekly e-news when registration opens each February. If you join through our affiliate group, I will invite you to our private *Birth Your Dreams* Facebook group where we not only learn from Marie valuable ways to market and grow our business, we will support each other as doulas and birth workers to vision and soar to new heights.

A book I also recommend is The Doula Business Guide: Creating a Successful MotherBaby Business.

Fees

Request at least partial payment as a retainer before starting the job. State in your written agreement, to be signed by your client, that this payment will be nonrefundable once your client has agreed to use your services after the initial home visit. The agreement is part of your prenatal questionnaire. A sample is provided at the end of chapter 2.

Most pregnant women can't remember anything. We joke that what little memory they have retained to the end of pregnancy is expelled with the placenta. Do not rely on a verbal agreement; your client won't remember it.

Once she has signed your agreement and paid her deposit, you are holding your time free for her. If she cancels, this may leave you without work that you turned away because you had a prior commitment to her. Chose a reasonable amount to charge as a nonrefundable deposit and include this information in your agreement. The balance for the initial package is due no later than your first day on the job after the birth. You may charge the same hourly rate all along or discount additional hours worked beyond the initial package.

A good minimum of time to plan for home visits is 16 hours, including the one-hour prenatal visit. You can choose to be flexible and start with fewer, it's your business, you can run it as you please. Remember, too, some clients will come to you in a flurry after the baby has already been born.

Every Friday, your client should pay for any additional hours that you worked that week. Aim for a minimum of three hours per day; often it is not worth the time to travel to a clients home for a shorter work session. Some doulas work a minimum of four hours per day, these details are up to you.

These decisions will be yours to make as you define your practice and rates. You might consider offering to spread out your hours over two weeks if other family members will be present and can help mom on certain days, many times families want the help of a doula even if grandparents will be around, let the family decide when they need you. In some cases you may not begin work until week two or three after delivery, when Dad has gone back to work and all family members have left. Women benefit from support throughout those first few weeks, so be flexible enough to meet each family's needs.

Some mothers may say that their partners will be at home during the first week, so they won't need you. You may want to point out that many families prefer to have your help even when both parents are home since many don't have experience with newborns or breastfeeding. You can suggest that, "Maybe I can come for a day or two to teach and support both of you and return when he or she returns to work and you will be alone with the baby."

People forget that having two or three adults around who don't know anything about newborn care is not much more useful than being alone. Knowledgeable support is essential for breastfeeding and very helpful in learning how to care for a newborn. In addition, you can provide help for the mom during her uncomfortable first week and be alert for any problems with the baby, such as jaundice.

Business Cards and Printed Promotional Materials

Presentation has become extremely important. Be able to create forms and letters on a computer, create a logo (or barter or pay someone to design one for you). It should be professional but friendly-just like you. Ask an artistic friend to design a logo in exchange for a day watching her child or a couple of dinners delivered to her door. If you know any graphic designers, they can be of tremendous help in designing your "business package." There are also many online services that can do this affordably. Use it for invoices, questionnaires, forms, and across your online presence. Using your logo on social media profiles will tie in to your website and present a cohesive brand.

Create a simple brochure that describes your services and fees. It doesn't have to be fancy, but should be perfectly spelled and look neat.

Business cards are essential as a networking and business tool. You'll enclose them when mailing your brochures and distribute them freely wherever you go. Post them on community and supermarket bulletin boards. Ask local shops, libraries, and bookstores if you may leave a stack in the appropriate section.

Deportment and Dress

Send an appropriate, clear message in everything you do. Act like the professional you are. If you are a smoker, don't smoke in your car on your way to your client's house. Nonsmokers pick up smoke on anything and may not let you in.

Perfume, too, is a no-no. Women are highly sensitive to smell. Some have respiratory problems that can cause them to have trouble breathing if even a light cologne is in the room. Sometimes people who have quit smoking become extremely sensitive to smell and feel ill in the presence of strong odors. To be safe, don't use fragrances at all.

Answer your business phone, even if it doubles as your home phone, in a professional manner and return calls promptly. Check your voice mail regularly (not while on a job). The message on your voice mail should be friendly and warm, not cute. It's best for your message to explain when the caller can expect a return call (such as, "I will call back within one business day"). Or state that you return calls between 8 and 9 p.m. or can be called until 9:30 p.m., whatever forks for you.

As a doula, you will temporarily act like a mother, sister, and friend. Dress like one. Being too dressed up is not practical for this work. On the other hand, should you dress in a way that is too relaxed or sloppy, or especially if your clothes are not clean, mom may not want you in her home or near her newborn. Even in jeans and a T-shirt, one person can look clean and neat and another, messy and dirty.

Some doulas like to wear doula T-shirts that they have bought at a doula conference or wear a special apron to cover their clothes. Take a spare clean shirt on every job, especially if you will go directly to another client after leaving the first.

As a doula you will cook, do light house cleaning, and care for mothers and newborns. These tasks call for flat, comfortable shoes that you can walk around and stand in for hours. Many families prefer you to remove your shoes when you arrive, keep a pair of slippers or shoes you only wear indoors in your doula bag. Always observe the family's standards and offer to remove your shoes while in their home. Select slippers that are snug fitting and not floppy, be sure they won't get caught going up and down stairs or pacing and rocking a baby.

Whatever you wear, make sure it's washable!

Marketing your Services

Clients change from month to month. You hope they will call again when they have their next baby, and many will, but that's likely to be two to four years away. Your referrals will tend to forget that you re out there unless you keep your name visible. Once you have developed a referral list, continue to market.

A Doula Speaks

I had been marketing our doula services to several area hospitals. One started to send us many referrals. I made it a point to call the nurse in charge to thank her. I asked if I could stop by and take her to breakfast or lunch. Nurses love offers of food no less than anyone else. She couldn't leave the hospital but met me in the cafeteria for breakfast one morning. I stayed in touch with her often as the referrals grew.

I decided that since we had established a great relationship, I could move on to develop connections with other hospitals. Four to six months went by and referrals from the original hospital dropped off. I had not called the nurse in a while, since I was busy doing other things. I had mistakenly assumed that our relationship didn't require ongoing maintenance.

One day at a meeting someone asked me if I still ran that doula service. She had seen the nurse I knew, who thought we might have gone out of business since she hadn't heard from me in a few months. What a shock! I learned my lesson: Marketing must be done all the time, even (or especially) with good referral sources.

Website

Even if you are just starting out, a website is a must. There are simple formats that you can do on your own with some computer skills, or find a designer who can help you get started and design the site for you. It is worth the initial expense as you must have an online presence and website for potential clients. Consider writing a blog to add to your website. There are many informative articles online to help guide you. Obtain and publish client testimonials on your website.

Paid Advertising

Paid advertising is probably not something you need to allocate a big portion of your budget to. There are many vehicles for marketing now that, when used effectively, can be a larger part of your marketing plan. However, be aware of print publications in which you'd like to be featured. Advertise in parenting papers or in appropriate organizations' directories with small ads that reproduce your business card. Take out ads in the Classified section of the local newspaper, ask for a special section called "Doulas." Look for local baby guides published by baby stores or other publications. Some newspapers will annually put out a special section for baby-related subjects. Find targeted publications that put your name in front of your target audience of pregnant families.

You can buy mailing lists of pregnant women in your region, separated by geography and economic status, and send them a flyer or brochure. Local printers such as the place that printed your brochures may know where the mailing houses that provide such lists are located. Print pretty gift certificates for your services and advertise them as baby shower presents.

Another form of paid advertising is to list your website or services on directory websites such as local online parents and baby guides or doula directories like Doula Match or All Doulas.

Social Media

Social media and networks are a great way to stay connected with past clients and to keep your name in the forefront for people searching for doulas. Always remember social media etiquette and confidentiality, never post about a client online unless they have given you express permission to do so. Even mentioning seemingly small, innocuous items sets a tone and can cross confidentiality lines. Instead post relevant articles, new studies, encouraging quotes or pictures, advertise a special event or a class.

Stay in touch with the people on your referral lists through social media messages, email and holiday and Mother's Day cards, sending a card on a baby's first birthday is another nice way to keep you in a family's mind. Generally, families with young babies are friends with others in that life stage and reminding them about you can help them refer you to a friend.

Press releases

Write one-page blurbs about anything newsworthy related to your business and email them to local newspapers. Contact local cable TV stations, too. Learn how to write a pitch and target it to the publication or media outlet you are contacting. For example, May is International Doula Month, write a release discussing what a doula is and the benefits of doula care, then close with your contact information and bio. You're giving the publication something of interest to their readers, they will not pick up an advertisement in the form of a press release.

Small newspapers are always looking for stories of local interest. When you first become a doula, submit a brief story about who you are, stating that you have recently completed your doula training and explaining what a doula does. Include a photograph. At the end of the article, include your telephone number and email for more information. This is free advertising, but be careful not to let it sound like an ad. Nevertheless, you can mention that gift certificates for doula services make an ideal gift at a baby shower or from a loving family member.

Press releases must be informational in content. A sample press release is provided at the end of this chapter. Send one every six months or whenever you have something new and different to say. You might ask a satisfied client if she would be willing to be interviewed about the work you did in her home. If she agrees, call a staff writer at the local paper and suggest that he or she interview her. Choose a client with an interesting situation, if you can, such as unexpected triplets.

Always look for new and different angles. Babies are popular subjects for photographs and the subject is so positive and family oriented that you can find ways to interest an editor.

Whenever new research comes out about doulas, contact the health editor of a larger paper and ask if she or he would like to report the research findings. Offer to serve as the local connection and to be interviewed.

Send local papers a press release after attending a major conference such as DONA International's, saying that a local doula has just returned from an international conference on doulas. List the speakers and their topics, new research of interest to the general public, and other pertinent information, again giving your name, website and contact information (and DONA International's) for people to follow up.

Networking

Seek out other doulas, online and local doula groups. Not only will doula contacts help with referrals, back up arrangements but they also help to discuss ideas and situations with others in the field. Gatherings to meet with other local doulas and workers in related fields should be frequent. Since much of this work is done in isolation, doulas need a place to recharge and share their good and bad experiences The more difficult the issues-high-risk populations with domestic violence, substance abuse, and low income, for example-the more important it is to have access to a support system to prevent burnout.

Record keeping

Whether you practice with a hospital or an agency or on your own, record keeping is essential. Agencies provide their own forms. A sample time sheet that you can use or adapt appears at the end of this chapter. Use one sheet for each client for each week. If you work for three clients in a given week, you will fill in three sheets that week. Carry these sheets in your doula notebook. Each day, record your hours and any special situations that occur. If all goes well, you can write a short general note listing what you have done for each family that week. If anything out of the ordinary occurs, write a more detailed account. Weeks or even days later you can easily forget details that might be important if anyone questioned you about what happened. When you have completed your work with a client, transfer those sheets to a larger notebook that you leave at home or in the office. To purchase online postpartum doula forms visit Birth Source

A Doula Speaks

More and more, I'm able to manage a doula client start to finish without paper. Using an iPad and apps like Evernote where I can keep records, notes, invoices and contracts all electronically. I enter every client into my phone, Dad or partner's phone number is listed as "other" within Mom's contact form and every meeting in my calendar is listed with the Mom's name first so it's easy to search my calendar for all of our visits to make invoicing simple. I also immediately insert the baby's birthday into my phone calendar with a yearly repeat reminder to send a first birthday card. Get creative and find ways to use technology to help you in your business.

Working for a Community-Based Agency

Being an employee of a community-based agency, of which many exist across North America, has many advantages. The agency will handle Social Security payments, worker's compensation, and other payroll obligations. The agency markets and advertises doula services, issues press releases, takes phone calls and emails, manages information and contracts with clients, and books the service.

Only after a client is committed to having a doula, with all the clerical work taken care of, will you receive her name and phone number. By then, the client will already understand the role of a doula, a big advantage, since you won't have to explain the basics of what you do to every potential client. The agency also handles all the bookkeeping, carries comprehensive liability insurance, bonds you against accidental breakage or theft, bills clients, and sends you your checks.

Don't underestimate the amount of time and money required to provide all the services listed above. To cover them, most agencies bill clients 50% more than the doula's wages.

Working with an agency gives your client a sense of reassurance as well. Hiring a doula through an agency assures her that she will be cared for with a certain level of professionalism. She knows that all the doulas who work for the agency are supervised and evaluated and that she will have recourse if a problem occurs.

Working for a Hospital-Based Doula Program

Many hospitals across the US are running their own doula programs, most are solely for labor support doulas, a few include postpartum doulas.

Birth is a natural, normal process. Until the 20th century, all births took place at home. Therefore, mothers and babies recovered in the comfort of their homes. Today, birth centers discharge women less than 24 hours after birth, and often 12 hours after birth, with excellent health and safety records. (See the Mother-Friendly Childbirth Initiative from the Coalition for Improving Maternity Services, reproduced following chapter 2, which contains a section on birth that relates to this issue.)

Many women who give birth in hospitals would prefer to rest, recover, and bond with their babies at home if they knew they would have help there. As a part of health care reform there is a new look at the role of the doula and the hope is that we will see an increase in hospital-based doula programs as well as community based doula programs that will provide postpartum doula care over one week or more, covered by Medicaid and other insurers.

For a doula, being a hospital employee has the same benefits as working for a community agency, doulas are often kept busier than they would be in independent practice or if they worked for a community agency. Community and independent doulas can experience high-volume and low-volume months, making work periods unpredictable. This inconsistent amount of work makes it difficult for many women to be doulas, especially if they need a guaranteed paycheck each week. The availability of work tends to follow the "feast-or-famine" model. Sometimes doulas work for two or three clients a week for months at a time. In contrast, when due dates fall late and client load is down, they may work for only a few hours a week or not at all, for weeks at a time.

Another advantage of working for a hospital-based service for the doula who wants to work most of the time is that hospitals may permit double shifts, so that she will visit one mother in the morning and another in the afternoon.

Hospital doula programs are often provided to women at no charge either because the services are covered by health insurance or because they are fully subsidized by the hospital. In areas where a high volume of mothers deliver and a hospital markets its doula service to all women during childbirth education classes and at providers' offices during prenatal visits, the proportion of birthing mothers who use the program ranges from 10% (usually for a new program) to 40%.

To find out if your local hospital has a doula program and how active it is, call the director of the doula program. If he hospital operator doesn't know what you're talking about, ask for the nurse in charge of postpartum care. If that doesn't work, ask for the maternity unit (not labor and delivery).

Ask how many births take place there each month and what proportion of birthing mothers use the service. Multiply these figures together to determine the approximate number of mothers who use the service each month. Ask how many doulas work for them full time and part time to find out how YOU would fit in.

Applying for a Job

Doula services that maintain a high standard of care hire only the best-qualified doulas. Applicants are asked to furnish personal information, which is kept on file confidentially.

In a high-quality service, doula selection requirements may include (but are not limited to) the items listed below. While having your own children and breast feeding experience would obviously be a great help, you don't personally have to have had every experience that a doula encounters. The service's final election will be based on personal interviews and appropriate recommendations. The interviewers "gut response" will play a big part, too. Some important issues:

- Your experiences and attitudes toward motherhood, babies, and children
- A penchant to be in the service of others
- A history of helping others
- Nurturing and parenting skills
- Breastfeeding experience
- Good health: free of communicable diseases, no substance abuse ("clean and sober"), negative tuberculosis test or a physician's note stating that you are not contagious (sometimes a person who has recovered from TB will test positive; a follow-up chest x-ray will demonstrate that she is clear of disease)
- Excellent interpersonal skills
- High school education or equivalent skills
- Receptiveness to learning new skills and information
- Demonstrated ability to make and keep commitments
- Availability to be present for five hours per day for home visits
- Knowledge of community resources
- Job experience in any area of maternal-child health, child development, or health care services.

You will probably be asked to provide up to three references from professionals, agencies, or organizations such as clergy, medical personnel, teachers, or officials of civic or community groups. You'll need these to provide to clients until you have accumulated references from clients themselves. Doulas should demonstrate their professionalism by offering references to clients without being asked.

Create a small binder in which you insert your resume/curriculum vitae (CV), references, a copy of your CPR certificate, copies of any training certificates, proof of attendance at workshops related to this work, proof of liability insurance, and any other relevant materials. (These are discussed in more detail below under "Establishing your credentials.") Take your binder to the initial home visit. Add the name and phone number of each client (with her permission) as you go along as references.

If you seem like a good prospect, you may be asked to think carefully about whether you have the appropriate qualifications to become a doula. How would you answer these typical interview questions:

Why do you want to be a doula?
What kinds of experience in your personal history will help you support families at this special time?
Tell me about the way your parents parented you.
If you have children, what things are you doing differently from the way your parents did them? Why?
If you are a mother, what do you like best about it?

Once hired, you will be expected to act professionally in every way. You will probably be given time sheets to fill out and submit to the head office. Hold the service to similarly professional standards. Expect ample warning about protocol changes and to be paid on time. Continuing education programs (there will be more on this later in this chapter) are extremely helpful; if they aren't offered, suggest that your agency start doing so.

One set of solutions is described later in this chapter in "How one doula service responded to staff stress."

Talk openly with the director of the service about any concerns. Tell her or him what's right, too.

Open communication should go both ways and constantly

Doula Bag Essentials and Options

Being professional means being prepared to introduce yourself and to provide safe, quality care. You will develop your own "bag of tricks" as you go on as a doula.

- Essentials
- Doula notebook.
- Copies of your references and evaluations
- A note, updated annually, from your health care provider stating that you are in good health to work with mothers and newborns

- Certificate of professional liability insurance
- Certificate from a doula training program
- Certification from a national or international organization that you have taken approved doula training and met certain criteria
- Card demonstrating that you have taken a course in infant/child CPR and first aid
- Time sheet for every current client
- Client's questionnaire and contact information as well as signed agreement and confidentiality agreement.
- GPS or a detailed map, printed detailed directions and/or a good road map of the area in which you work will help you get around. Don't get lost! Plan your route the night before.
- Box of disposable surgical gloves. You will need these for diaper changes and laundry. You can buy these at most pharmacies and medical supply companies. If you have skin allergies or are allergic to latex, buy what's appropriate for you. Otherwise, buy whatever is on sale.
- A clean shirt. Babies spit up and spills happen, so be prepared. Some doulas choose to wear a smock. You might have a special doula shirt printed with your logo. Otherwise pack an extra shirt and layers depending upon how warm/cool clients keep their home, you can adjust your clothing to your comfort.
- List of professional referrals. These are related professionals to whom you may wish to refer your clients, such as other doulas, lactation consultants, and nurse-midwives. Keep copies of those professionals' brochures and/or business cards to give to clients as needed. As you travel around to market your services, collect brochures from related services. If a mom would like to join a postpartum exercise class or learn infant massage, you can help her decide where to go.
- First aid manual. You'll get one at your first aid course.

Options

Choose what you find useful.

- Massage lotions, oils or tools. You might take a bottle of unscented massage lotion and a bottle of lavender or jasmine lotion; both promote relaxation.
- Aromatherapy oils. Consider exploring this growing field, which acknowledges that we are affected by all our senses. Smell is one that we often ignore. We can use these concepts to help women relax; jasmine and lavender are recommended for relaxation if the mother likes them, always be sure to check with mom's preferences and allergies.
- Recordings of soothing music. See the section "Soothing music for relaxation" at the end of chapter 4.
- Samples of Lansinoh cream. Great for sore nipples, this cream is available from lactation consultants and drugstores. You can get free tiny samples attached to useful brochures on breast feeding by contacting Lansinoh and saying you're a doula.

- Personal items such as medications or vitamins. You may need these to keep your strength up. You never know what kind of day you'll have. Bring any personal care items you might need.

- Books for siblings. For more on this, see chapter 9, "Offering support to the new mother's family."

Professional Development and Networking

Doulas typically work in isolation. Postpartum is a vast field, as you have already seen from the many topics covered in previous chapters, yet we have been able only to reveal briefly what a postpartum doula may see in a given year. Postpartum doulas are generalists, we need to have a good understanding on a broad range of topics.

To continue learning, doulas need to attend continuing education workshops, conferences and to participate in networking opportunities. They need emotional support and sharing time with other doulas, too. Many issues can be extremely difficult to cope with on your own and it helps to have strong support from experienced doulas.

A Doula Speaks

In the early days of marriage, my husband sat and listened in fascination to every detail of my work. Now he says, "Did she have a boy or girl? Is she breastfeeding? Great; all is well." He really is tired of hearing my descriptions of sore, cracked nipples or a new mom's lack of sleep, yet I often still need to share those stories.

That's where my doula friends come in. Whether the day has been great or stressed and difficult, having other doulas available for "de-briefing" is important.

Continuing Education

You must learn about your obligation, according to your own state laws, to report child abuse and what to do if you come upon it. You need to know about resources for domestic violence and issues that are associated with it. One in four women is sexually abused in her lifetime. That experience frequently plays into feelings about delivery and motherhood. Penny Simkin's book, *When Survivor's Give Birth*, is essential reading for doulas, and visit PATTCh, Prevention and Treatment of Traumatic Childbirth for resources and information.

Often childbirth is a "trigger time" when memories and issues from past abuse flood to the surface. They can confuse and alter the woman's feelings about her body and her baby. Attending a workshop on this topic or doing additional reading and sharing your findings and experiences at an in-service program or networking session is very important.

Other excellent topics for continuing education include drug and alcohol abuse, adult and infant massage, group meditations, and herbs and other healing alternatives for postpartum women. Valerie

Lynn's book *The Mommy Plan, Restoring Your Post-Pregnancy Body Naturally, Using Women's Traditional Wisdom* is a good book to start if you would like to learn more about traditional baths and postpartum nurturing practices. Consider inviting any or all of the following as guest speakers: pediatricians, midwives, nurse practitioners, and lactation consultants. An obstetrician might answer common questions, discuss his or her practice, and provide a great marketing opportunity for the doulas who attend.

Working as a postpartum doula in people's homes raises many issues. The more we learn, the more we realize how little we know. Attending workshops locally, nationally and internationally as well as, workshops from providers in your community is an excellent way to acquire knowledge and another way to network.

Ask local providers to bring your group a presentation on what they do for new mothers, fathers or families. Help them educate you about when and how to make an appropriate referral to them. For example, when should you call in a lactation consultant and when can you as a doula handle a breastfeeding problem on your own? What do their services include? How much do they charge? Are they available to you for a free phone consultation to talk over a client's simple problem before making a home visit?

Learn about working with women and alcohol or substance abuse. Find out about community referrals. Study child abuse. The reach of your continuing education will depend on the community you serve and how you define the scope of your practice.

If your hospital or agency is not providing such programs, or if you are working independently, consider forming your own education group and keep one another informed of local workshops to increase your knowledge and keep you up to date. Ask childbirth educators, La Leche League leaders, other doulas, and even interested clients to arrange for guest speakers. Such meetings provide fine opportunities for sharing the joys and challenges of your careers and developing a referral system

All these topics are too complex for us to cover in this manual.

Creating Doula Outreach and Support Groups

Many doulas are starting independent networks in which a group of doulas, often including both birth doulas and postpartum doulas, get together and formally found an organization. These groups write mission statements and membership policies and cooperate to market, educate, and support doulas in their regions. By working together, doulas can maintain their independence while sharing efforts to promote, educate, mentor, and expand doula services in their communities.

Co-author Debra Pascali-Bonaro is involved with BirthNet, a network of independent doulas and childbirth educators of northern New Jersey and Rockland County, New York. BirthNet maintains a speaker's bureau and offers various levels of membership. There are subcommittees on public relations, mentoring, membership, and education. Research if you have an existing Birth Network or MotherBaby Network in your region, and if not consider starting one. Visit Birth Network as well as IMBCI.

Networking is like fast food: The more chains spring up in one region, the better they all do. The more doulas we have, the more women will know about us, choose to use us, and tell their friends and neighbors about us. Rather than competing with each other, doulas should share a sense of community and learn to nurture each other. Not every doula will be right for every family.

The following story illustrates why we should work together. We found this gem on the Internet. We don't know where it came from, but hope that whoever wrote it will be pleased to have it reproduced here.

A Sense of a Goose

Next fall, when you see geese heading south for the winter, consider what science has discovered about why they fly that way.

As each bird flaps its wings, it creates uplift for the bird immediately following. By flying in "V" formation, the whole flock adds at least 71 % greater flying range than if each bird flew on its own.

People who share a common direction and sense of community can get where they are going more quickly and easily because they are traveling on the thrust of one another.

When a goose falls out of formation, it suddenly feels the drag and resistance of trying to go it alone and quickly gets back into formation to take advantage of the lifting power of the bird in front.

If we have as much sense as a goose, we will stay in formation with those people who are headed the same way we are. When the head goose gets tired, it rotates back in the wing and another goose flies point. It is sensible to take turns doing demanding jobs. Geese honk from behind to encourage those up front to keep up their speed. What messages do we give when we honk from behind?

When a goose gets sick or is wounded by gunshot and falls out of formation, two other geese fall out with that goose and follow it down to lend help and protection. They stay with the fallen goose until it is able to fly or it dies. Only then do they launch out on their own or join another formation in an effort to catch up with their own group. If we have the sense of a goose, we will stand by each other like that.

Whatever model of doula care you choose to work in, maintain a group of other doulas who can provide backup for you (and you for them) as needed. Enlist the support not only of one other doula but also of her backup. If you develop a slight cold or worse, you can't go into the home of a newborn. A family emergency or the surprise of having two clients give birth at the same time may also prevent you from fulfilling all your doula obligations.

The families you serve will count on you. Be clear about your role, scope of practice, and availability. It is fine to state your limitations on when you can work for them, but make sure that whatever you mutually agree to, you can uphold. Connecting informally with a group or more formally with a partner is essential for all doulas.

A Doula Tale: How One Doula Service Responded to Staff Stress

Being in a service role is a time of learning as well as sharing. When a doula works in difficult situations, she needs a place to go where she can share her experiences, but also feel supported herself. Many doulas internalize emotions and feel stressed when they don't have access to a support system. That's one benefit of working for a community group/agency that plans regular in-service workshops. Other options are finding doulas in your area and meeting to support one another, you could organize birth sharing circles in which client's confidentiality is maintained but doulas are able to talk and help process difficult births or help one another learn and grow from their experiences.

In the mid-1990s, Debra Pascali-Bonaro expanded her doula service to direct a community based doula program in inner city Paterson, New Jersey, called the Neighborhood Doula Project (described in "Why we became doulas: reflections by the authors" near the beginning of this manual). The program served pregnant women in recovery from substance abuse, alcohol addiction, or both. Suddenly the doulas were dealing with women who were coping with inadequate housing, insufficient food and clothing, domestic violence, issues of past sexual abuse, and addiction.

To prevent instant burnout, the doulas met weekly for three hours to discuss the difficulties their clients faced and to work together to find solutions. Periodically they used workshop time to nurture themselves and each other. They used meditations, healing ceremonies, and prayer to accommodate the life situations they were observing at first hand, most of them for the first time. Building in this time for doulas to share, learn and grow is essential to our personal development and well-being.

Joining National Organizations and Attending Conferences

National groups can help you learn about many aspects of being a postpartum doula, they can help you make connections in the doula field and connect you with supportive resources and forums. The following organizations are recommended for networking, certifying, publications, and conferences:

- DONA International
- Common Sense Childbirth Perinatal Outreach
- Childbirth and Postpartum Professional Association (CAPPA)
- Health Connect One
- Full Circle Doulas
- International Childbirth Education Association (ICEA)
- Doula Trainings International (DTI)
- Childbirth International
- Academy of Certified Birth Educators and Labor Support Professionals

Sample application form
for a postpartum doula

Dimple Doula Services, Inc.

1535 Baby St.
Newborn, IN 46000
Phone: (555) 555-5555
Fax: (555) 555-5556
Email: dimpledoula@baby.com
www.dimpledoula.com

Name: _____

Address: _____

Contact number: _____

Email: _____

Age: _____

Social Security Number: _____

Employment history (most recent first):

1.

2.

3.

Formal education (degrees, certification):

_____

Other related education (workshops, classes, or conferences attended that are related to postpartum care): _____

Related life experience (include a brief description of childbirth and breastfeeding experience); use back of sheet, if necessary: _____

Do you have a favorite cooking style, such as vegetarian, whole foods, Italian, or Japanese? _____

Are you comfortable trying other cooking styles? _____

Do you smoke? _____

Do you have reliable transportation? _____

Automobile insurance company and policy number: _____

Work availability (mornings, afternoons, both? specific hours?): _____

Three references (please do not include relatives): _____

Name Address Contact Number Occupation Relationship to you

1. _____

2. _____

3. _____

Do you have a criminal record? Yes No

If yes, please explain: _____

Have you been, or are you now, involved as a defendant in any investigation, hearing, disciplinary action, or claim? If you are, please explain: _____

Why do you want to do this work? _____

Signature & Date: _____

Sample thank-you letter
to client after completing job

(accompanies client evaluation form)
Dimple Doula Services, Inc.

1535 Baby St.
Newborn, IN 46000
Phone: (555) 555-5555
Fax: (555) 555-5556
Email: dimpledoula@baby.com
www.dimpledoula.com

March 15, 2014

Sally Marner
2828 New England Dr.
Wharton, MN 55556

Dear Sally:

I am writing to thank you for using Dimple Doula Services. I hope that our staff was able to meet your needs during your first weeks with your new baby. If we can be of any further assistance to you, please do not hesitate to call.

We have established a reference file for future clients as well as for our own information and would appreciate your comments. I know how busy you are, but I would really appreciate it if you could take a few moments to fill in our evaluation form.

Many health insurance companies are reimbursing families for part or all of the fee for postpartum doula care. Your receipt is for your medical records. We suggest that you request reimbursement from your health insurance carrier, attaching a copy of this receipt and the carrier's claim form. To increase your chances of reimbursement, include a prescription from your physician or midwife for our services, if possible.

Besides gaining reimbursement for yourself, encouraging insurance companies to recognize the importance of this type of service will help new mothers in the future. If we can help you to process the claim, please contact us.

We appreciate your taking the time to fill out the enclosed evaluation form. A selfaddressed stamped envelope is enclosed for your convenience.

Thank you for letting us "mother" you and allowing us to be a part of such a special time in your life.

With warm wishes,

(Your name/company)

Sample client evaluation form

Dimple Doula Services, Inc.

1535 Baby St.
Newborn, IN 46000
Phone: (555) 555-5555
Fax: (555) 555-5556
Email: dimpledoula@baby.com
www.dimpledoula.com

Name: _____

Address: _____

Contact number: _____

Email: _____

1. Did our service: (please mark one):

Meet your expectations? Exceed your expectations? Fall short of your expectations?

2. How well did Dimple Doula Services, Inc., meet your needs in the following areas? (please check only one rating for each category)

Excellent, Good, Fair, Poor, or N/A

    Mothercare
    Family care
    Newborn care
    Breastfeeding support
    Cooking
    Tidying
    Laundry
    Shopping/Errands
    Other (specify)

3. Were you comfortable having [insert doulas name] work for you? Yes/No

4. What was the most helpful part of our service? _____

5. What was the least helpful part of our service? _____

6. Were you happy with the length of service? Yes/No

7. Did having a doula affect your decision or ability to breastfeed? Yes/No

Please comment about how a doula affected your breastfeeding experience: _____

8. Would you recommend the service to other families? Yes/No

9. May we give your name and phone number to other clients for reference? Yes/No

10. Please add any additional comments: _____

11. Names and contact information of friends or family members who might like to receive our brochure (use back of page for additional space if needed): _____

Sample press release

When writing press releases, imagine that you are an average person reading the article in a local newspaper. Don't use clinical terms such as "postpartum." Do use short sentences and short paragraphs.

Format: At the top of the page, include the date, "FOR IMMEDIATE RELEASE," and "Contact:," followed by your name and daytime phone number, in case the recipient has questions. You never know-you may trigger an interview or a big feature story.

Double space. If you need a second sheet (never use the back), repeat the date and contact information at the top and say "Doula story, page 2 of 2."

Style: Write in third-person newspaper style. "I" becomes "she." "You" is not used.

Write a simple newspaper-style headline that summarizes the story. Use the present tense without "is" or "are" ("Doula opens practice in Diapertown") or use the future tense, with an infinitive ("Doula to open practice in Diapertown").

Put the most important information early in the story. Newspapers often cut from the end.

DIMPLE DOULA SERVICES, INC.

1535 Baby St.
Newborn, IN 46000
Phone: (555) 555-5555 Fax: (555) 555-5556
Email: dimpledoula@baby.com
www.dimpledoula.com

FOR IMMEDIATE RELEASE March 15, 2014 CONTACT: (Your name and daytime phone number)

Local Doula Can "Mother the Mother" After Childbirth

Pregnancy, birth and the early weeks at home with a new baby are exciting times. They're also busy and sometimes confusing and overwhelming times, when families need a tremendous amount of support and information.

Doulas, a new addition to our maternity care system, recreate the woman-to-woman network of the past. They represent a return to the traditional ways of "mothering the mother."

The Greek word "doula" (DOO-la) means "a woman who serves." Most doulas have children of their own and are keenly aware of how sensitive and vulnerable a woman feels during pregnancy, labor, birth and the early weeks as a new mother.

A doula first visits the mother during pregnancy. After the birth, she comes to the house to provide instruction on taking care of the new mother after delivery and her newborn, including breastfeeding or bottle-feeding. She assists with siblings, cooking, laundry and general care of the family and home. She does not provide medical care.

Doula programs are gaining in popularity nationwide. Some insurance carriers pay for doulas for all their maternity patients if they choose to leave the hospital within 24 hours of giving birth. [If that's true of a hospital in your area, say so.]

[Your name], who recently graduated from a rigorous doula training course, is now caring for new mothers in the area. Anyone who would like to learn more about doulas may contact [your name] at [your phone number]. An excellent source of nationwide referrals is DONA International www.dona.org

Sample time sheet and client report

If you work for an agency, you will probably be given forms like this to keep track of the hours you have worked and what you have done for each client. Each form represents one week of work for one client. If you work for yourself or your agency doesn't provide such forms, keep a journal to track the same information. You may need it later or simply wish to refer to it for many reasons. The journal doesn't have to be fancy. A simple spiral-bound notebook from a stationery store is fine.

DIMPLE DOULA SERVICES, INC.

1535 Baby St.
Newborn, IN 46000
Phone: (555) 555-5555
Fax: (555) 555-5556
Email: dimpledoula@baby.com
www.dimpledoula.com

TIME SHEET AND EMPLOYEE REPORT

Week of: _____

Branch manager: _____

Name of doula: _____

Address: _____

Client name: _____

Address: _____

Home Phone: _____

Cell Phone: _____

Email: _____

Date Day of Week Hours: _____

TOTAL HOURS WORKED: _____

Employee Report

Briefly describe the services that you provided to this client, including if you provided education, referral, nurturing, or list the type of support for each type of care.

Mother care: _____

Breastfeeding support: _____

Newborn care: _____

Cooking: _____

Sibling care: _____

Laundry: _____

Light housekeeping: _____

Other: _____

Sample marketing letter

Dimple Doula Services, Inc.

1535 Baby St.
Newborn, IN 46000
Phone: (555) 555-5555
Fax: (555) 555-5556
Email: dimpledoula@baby.com
www.dimpledoula.com

March 15, 2014

Olympia Orange, R.N., M.5.N.
Director of Nursing and Related Services
Thor Hospital, "W" Wing, 3rd Floor 1447 Cloud St.
Valhalla, IN 47000

Dear Ms. Orange:

Thank you for taking the time to review the enclosed materials on our perinatal services. We hope you will consider recommending Dimple Doula Services, Inc., to women who give birth at your facility. Our approach is not primarily to take care of the baby but to "mother the mother," her partner, and their family and to support them in their new role, starting with pregnancy and continuing through labor, birth, and the first weeks postpartum.

Dimple Doula Services, Inc., is dedicated to nurturing the new mother and partner so that they can more easily bond with and nurture their baby We accomplish this by providing emotional support and encouragement as well as instruction in newborn care and breastfeeding. We do not attempt to provide medical care or advice but may suggest that mom call her provider, if appropriate. We lend a hand with household tasks such as grocery shopping, tending to an older sibling, doing the dishes, cooking simple meals, and handing mom a cup of tea.

Our initial package includes a one-hour prenatal interview in the client's home followed by 15 hours of postpartum home care. The doula who will work with the family visits the home to discuss what is needed and to explain what she can do.

Hours are flexible and based on each client's needs. Most clients choose to have the doula visit for three hours per day for five days. The maximum a doula works on a given day is five hours. Our rate is $__ per hour. Additional hours may be purchased beyond the initial package. Gift certificates are available.

We have been talking with insurance companies and hospitals about the possibility of third-party reimbursement for doula services and would be happy to work with you in this effort, if you are interested.

A booklet describing our services and a sample of our client questionnaire for postpartum care are enclosed. We would be glad to send our literature to anyone on request. Please call if you would like any additional information or to arrange a personal meeting.

Sincerely,

(Your name)

Suggested Reading:

DONA Postpartum Reading List
DONA Birth Doula Reading List

Welcome!

You couldn't wait, Small, smallest in-a-hurry
Son #3, impatient to see what
Your brothers had in store (ah, not to worry,
They'd plotted, planned their mischief), you forgot
What day it was, that you'd not been invited
To join the pair until - why, weeks from now!
We thought you'd come for lunch. We were excited
About welcoming. We'd show you how
A family full of boys would tease another,
Would give a noisy shout, would laugh and cheer
And share a father further, and a mother.
You came for breakfast! Littlest and dear
Beyond these giddy words, we're glad you're here.

- Maureen Cannon

RESOURCES

Debra's Web Sites

www.debrapascalibonaro.com- To learn more about Debra's workshops, webinars, and conferences where she will be speaking around the world, as well as to join her weekly wisdom.

www.orgasmicbirth.com- Debra Pascali-Bonaro is producer and director of the films Orgasmic Birth and Organic Birth, two films documenting the sensual and life changing aspects of undisturbed childbirth as well as co-author of the book: *Orgasmic Birth: Your Guide to A Safe, Satisfying and Pleasurable Birth Experience.*

Please join me on www.facebook.com/obirth as well as join my e-newsletter to learn more about special offers, upcoming webinars and advanced retreats.

Pregnancy and Birth

Childbirth Connection A source for trustworthy up-to-date evidence-based information and resources on planning for pregnancy, labor, and birth and the postpartum period, promoting safe, effective, satisfying evidence-based maternity care for women and families and their Transform Childbirth Connection site.

Mother's Advocate Videos and handouts to create a safe and healthy birth.

Positions for Labor Great Handouts

Acupressure for Labor and Birth Great You Tube images

Booklet of Natural Pain Relief Techniques

Coalition for Improving Maternity Services The Mother-Friendly Childbirth Initiative provides guidelines for identifying "mother-friendly" birth sites, including hospitals, birth centers, and homebirth services in the U.S. Many great handouts and information on induction, cesarean birth and "10 questions to ask" brochure.

International MotherBaby Childbirth Initiative The purpose of the IMBCI 10 Steps is to improve care throughout the childbearing continuum in order to save lives, prevent illness and harm from the overuse of obstetric technologies, and promote health for mothers and babies around the world.

Mothers Naturally Goal: to increase the number of safe and positive births by educating and informing the public about natural birth options and empowering women to make pregnancy and birth choices appropriate for their lives. A public education program from the Midwives Alliance of North America (see under Midwifery).

Our Bodies Ourselves (OBOS) Also known as the *Boston Women's Health Book Collective* (BWHBC), is a nonprofit, public interest women's health education, advocacy, and consulting organization. Beginning in 1970 with the publication of the first edition of Our Bodies, Ourselves, OBOS has inspired the women's health movement and their books and resources are a must read for all women!

March of Dimes Mission is to help moms have full-term pregnancies and research the problems that threaten the health of babies.

Preeclampsia Foundation The Preeclampsia Foundation is an empowered community of patients and experts, with a diverse array of resources and support to help you have the best possible pregnancy or to help you navigate the questions you'll have if you don't. We provide unparalleled support and advocacy for the people whose lives have been or will be affected by the condition - mothers, babies, fathers and their families.

Sidelines - National High Risk Pregnancy Support Sidelines is a 501 ©(3) non-profit organization providing international support for women and their families experiencing complicated pregnancies and premature births. We believe that families can cope more successfully with a high-risk pregnancy with appropriate medical intervention, education, and a strong support system.

Planned Parenthood Planned Parenthood believes in the fundamental right of each individual, throughout the world, to manage his or her fertility, regardless of the individual's income, marital status, race, ethnicity, sexual orientation, age, national origin, or residence.

Spinning Babies Babies settle in the easiest position they can for birth. A good fetal position helps the cervix open more easily and labor progress smoothly. *Mother's job is to dilate; Baby's job is to rotate.*

International Cesarean Awareness Network www.ican-online.org Formed more than 25 years ago to support women in their journey toward understanding the risks of cesarean section and to help them have healthy births and healthy lives after undergoing the surgery that changed them. Great resources and tips for all women who are birthing in facilities with high cesarean birth rates.

VBAC (vaginal birth after cesarean)

VBAC.COM

Provides access to information from scientific studies, professional guidelines, government reports, successful and safe established VBAC programs, and the midwifery model of care with the goal of helping women make informed decisions about how they will give birth and to encourage an honest and respectful dialog with their caregivers.

VBAC Facts The mission of VBAC Facts is simple: to make hard-to-find, interesting, and pertinent information relative to post-cesarean birth options easily accessible to the people who seek it.

Childbirth Education

Active Birth Centre Provides information on the active birth programme with waterbirth, pregnancy, and professional training. Also has a free e-journal and products for sale. London

Bradley Method of Natural Childbirth Bradley classes stress the importance of healthy baby, healthy mother, and healthy families, attracting families who are willing to take the responsibility needed for preparation and birth.

HypnoBirthing® The Mongan Method is a unique method of relaxed, natural childbirth education, enhanced by self-hypnosis techniques. HypnoBirthing® provides the missing link that allows women to use their natural instincts to bring about a safer, easier, more comfortable birthing. Emphasis is placed on pregnancy and childbirth, as well as on pre-birth parenting and the consciousness of the pre-born baby.

Birthing From Within Birthing From Within gave us a chance to deeply and authentically explore our pre-conceived notions, fears, hopes, and dreams about birth and new parenthood.

Childbirth International A worldwide community of doulas, childbirth educators, and breastfeeding counselors.

International Childbirth Education Association Freedom of choice based on knowledge of alternatives in family-centered maternity and newborn care.

Lamaze International Promotes, supports, and protects normal birth through education and advocacy. View new Safe Birth practice videos.

National Childbirth Trust British charity informs and supports parents through pregnancy, birth, and the early days of parenthood.

Birth Works Birth is instinctive... Birth Works believes that the knowledge about how to give birth is born within every woman. Therefore, birth is instinctive and what is instinctive doesn't need to be taught. Birth Works helps women to have more trust and faith in their own body knowledge that already knows how to give birth. This is a unique approach that is empowering and transforming in nature.

Consumer Groups

BOLD is a global arts-based movement inspiring communities to create childbirth choices that work for mothers through performances of the play Birth and BOLD Red Tents around the world.

Birth Networks have formed independently in at least nine states as well as in Canada and Australia.

These grassroots community organizations promote normal birth; endorse the Mother-Friendly Childbirth Initiative; provide support, education, and evidenced-based information about normal birth for parents; and serve as a resource for caregivers who support normal birth.

The Birth Survey is a mechanism for women to share information about maternity care practices in their communities and a source of feedback to practitioners and institutions toward improving quality of care.

Citizens for Midwifery Works to provide information and resources that promote the local midwife as well as midwives and midwifery care nationwide. The only national consumer-based group in the United States promoting the Midwives Model of Care.

Human Rights

Amnesty International *Demand Dignity - Deadly Delivery Report.* It's more dangerous to give birth in the United States than in 49 other countries. African-American women are at almost four times greater risk than Caucasian women. A safe pregnancy is a human right for every woman regardless of race or income.

The White Ribbon Alliance is leading change from grassroots to global level, making needless maternal deaths a thing of the past.

Respectful Care in Childbirth

Human Rights in Childbirth Every health care system in the world faces the same essential questions. Who decides how a baby is born? Who chooses where a birth takes place? Who bears the ultimate responsibility for a birth and its outcome? What are the legal rights of birthing women? What are the responsibilities of doctors, midwives and other caregivers in childbirth? What are the rights and interests of the unborn, and how are they protected?

Doulas

DONA International The oldest and largest doula association in the world serves mothers and families by providing access to information and research about doulas, childbirth, and the postpartum experience.

The Prison Birth Project The Prison Birth Project (PBP) is a reproductive justice organization providing support, education, advocacy, and activism training to women at the intersection of the criminal justice system and motherhood. In prison, 4-7% of women are pregnant, the same percentage as in the wider population; 85% are mothers, and 25% were pregnant upon arrest or gave birth in the previous year.

The Doula Project The Doula Project is an NYC-based organization that provides free compassionate care and emotional, physical, and informational support to people across the spectrum of pregnancy.

YourDoulaBiz.com is designed by a doula for doulas. Manage your all of your client data from contact information to birth preferences and all data in between. Setup tasks such as interviews and prenatal appointments. Keep track of mileage and expenses for appointments. Quickly and easily email client data to your backup doula(s)

Doula Match Marketing of your doula services

Midwifery

Midwives Alliance of North America A professional organization for all midwives with the goal of unifying and strengthening the profession of midwifery.

The National Association of Certified Professional Midwives (NACPM) A professional association committed to significantly increasing women's access to quality maternity care by supporting the work and practice of Certified Professional Midwives.

American College of Nurse-Midwives Mission: to promote the health and well-being of women and infants within their families and communities through the development and support of the profession of midwifery as practiced by certified nurse-midwives and certified midwives.

Foundation for the Advancement of Midwifery Fulfills its mission-to improve the health status of women, babies, and families by increasing awareness of and access to the midwifery model of care-by funding education, research, and public policy initiatives.

International Confederation of Midwives Supports, represents, and works to strengthen professional associations of midwives; works with midwives and midwifery associations globally to secure women's right and access to midwifery care before, during, and after childbirth.

Midwifery Today Quarterly journal written mostly by midwives, doctors, doulas, childbirth educators, academics, and other specialists; sponsors worldwide midwifery conferences.

AABC - American Association of Birth Centers We are a multi-disciplinary membership organization comprised of individuals and organizations who support the birth center concept. Birth Centers uphold the rights of healthy women and their families, in all communities, to birth their children in an environment which is safe, sensitive and cost effective with minimal intervention.

Breastfeeding

La Leche League International Gives information and encouragement to mothers who want to breast-feed their babies, recognizing the unique importance of one mother helping another to perceive the needs of her child and to learn the best means of fulfilling those needs.

World Alliance for Breastfeeding Action A global network of individuals and organizations concerned with the protection, promotion, and support of breastfeeding worldwide.

At Breastfeeding Inc., our aim is to empower parents by ensuring they receive the most up-to-date information to assist them with their breastfeeding baby. We strive to provide them this information through breastfeeding resources which include, but are not limited to, free information sheets, video clips, and articles. Some resources, such as books, protocols and videos can also be purchased through the website.

The Breast Crawl: A Scientific Overview Every newborn, when placed on her mother's abdomen, soon after birth, has the ability to find her mother's breast all on her own and to decide when to take the first breastfeed. This is called the 'Breast Crawl'.

ILCA - International Lactation Consultant Association The International Lactation Consultant Association(tm) (ILCA(tm)) is the professional association for International Board Certified Lactation Consultants® (IBCLC®) and other health care professionals who care for breastfeeding families. ILCA membership is open to all who support and promote breastfeeding; you can join at anytime and do not need to be an IBCLC to become a member.

Office on Women's Health, U.S. Department of Health and Human Services

Parenting

Fathers-To-Be provides information, education, forums and products for parents and childbirth professionals worldwide.

Fatherhood Institute UK's Fatherhood Think Tank. Best resource for research on fathers and the family.

Mindful Mama is a community of moms and the people who love them. Visit often to read up on mindful approaches to pregnancy, adoption, birth, and parenting.

Mothering Magazine includes both evidence-based clinical articles and articles written by parents, all supporting simple and natural parenting and living.

National Association of the Mothers of Twins Clubs, Inc. was founded in 1960 for the purpose of promoting the special aspects of child development which relate specifically to multiple birth children.

ZERO TO THREE is a national, nonprofit organization that informs, trains, and supports professionals, policymakers, and parents in their efforts to improve the lives of infants and toddlers.

Waterbirth

Waterbirth International Great site for Workshops and Waterbirth Information and research.

Birth Balance Equipment, protocols, books, movies, photos, birth stories. The East Coast USA waterbirth resource center since 1987.

Sheila Kitzinger's waterbirth page A collection of resources and information about waterbirth from the well-known British birth activist.

Waterbirth Solutions Waterbirth Solutions is the US distributor for the Aquaborn Eco Birth Pool as well as the exclusive distributor for the high quality, unique and affordable permanent hospital tubs which were designed by Barbara Harper the founder of Waterbirth International.

Birth Equipment Birth tubs and birth stools.

Circumcision

National Organization of Circumcision Information Resource Centers

Jewish Birth Network: A Gray Area Guide to the Circumcision Debate July, 2011 Blog Post by Rabbi Shira Shazeer

Postpartum Resources

Prevention and Treatment of Traumatic Childbirth - PATTCh is a collective of birth and mental health experts dedicated to the prevention and treatment of traumatic childbirth.

Birth Trauma Association UK-based group offers emotional and practical support to women who have had a traumatic birth experience and their families.

Solace for Mothers is an organization designed for the sole purpose of providing and creating support for women who have experienced childbirth as traumatic. Birth trauma is real and can result from an even seemingly "normal" birth experience.

Robyn's Nest Post Traumatic Stress Disorder After Childbirth Provides educational information and support for women who have experienced PTSD after childbirth or related disorders.

Trauma and Birth Stress New Zealand-based organization focuses on posttraumatic stress disorder as a result of a traumatic birth experience.

Postpartum Support International is dedicated to helping women suffering from perinatal mood and anxiety disorders, including postpartum depression, the most common complication of childbirth. We also work to educate family, friends and healthcare providers so that moms and moms-to-be can get the support they need and recover.

Postpartum DADS This website is intended to help dads and families by providing firsthand information and guidance through the experience of PPD. This site also includes information and resources that can be used by professionals to assist families dealing with PPD.

Healthy Families America Healthy Families America, a program of PCA America, strives to provide all expectant and new parents with the opportunity to receive the education and support they need at the time their baby is born.

Grief and Loss:

Please refer to Chapter 10 Unexpected Outcomes for many grief, loss and special needs resources.

Business Resources:

The Doula Business Guide to Creating a Successful MotherBaby Business, by Patti Brennan

Creating and Marketing Your Birth Related Business, by Connie Livingston and her daughter Heather Livingston

The Small Business Administration

SCORE is a non-profit association dedicated to helping small businesses get-off the ground, grow and achieve their goals through education and mentorship. Because our work is supported by the U.S. Small Business Administration (SBA), and thanks to our network of 13,000+ volunteers, we are able to deliver our services at no charge or at very low cost.

Cutting Edge Press Cutting Edge Press was founded in 1994 in Houston, Texas. CEP provided a forum for "cutting edge" books concerning childbirth. We have served the healthcare industry for more than 10 years by providing the widest range possible of "cutting edge" books and other maternity care products.

Childbirth Graphics Teaching tools for healthcare and birth professionals.

Birth Source Perinatal Education Associates is an international company dedicated to promoting positive pregnancy outcomes through education, promotion of evidence-based research, family centered care, maternal/child health advocacy and awareness.

Your Doula Bag Doula resources and business support

March of Dimes Tools for Professionals. The March of Dimes campaign, "Healthy Babies Are Worth the Wait," aims to raise awareness about the critical development that occurs during the last few weeks of pregnancy and dispel the myth that it's safe to schedule a delivery before 39 weeks of pregnancy without a medical need. The website offers general information about the campaign as well as a "Less than 39 weeks" toolkit for professionals.

Using Technology for Your Birth Business

If you haven't yet taken your birth business online, you're missing out. If you run an independent childbirth education, doula or midwifery business, maintaining a website and participating in social media are essential components to competing and succeeding in today's market.

For creating your website, check out these five inexpensive (or free!) website building options with ready-made designs and layouts reviewed in this article on Mashable. For tips on effective social media use, check out the informative article on Science & Sensibility, Making Healthy Birth Go Viral: Why Birth Professionals Should Be on Social Media.

A Path to Good Doula/Midwife/Medical Professional Relationships

Read more about research on doula programs in The First Days of Life: Adding Doulas to Early Childhood Programs by the Ounce of Prevention Fund.

Research Resources

The Birth Facts Evidence based information organized by topic. Includes a selection of free handouts for use in your practice.

PubMed Large database of published studies, literature reviews, etc. The site also includes a great section of tutorials on how to search for and find the topics you are interested in.

The Cochrane Collaboration Large collection of systemic reviews on a wide variety of topics. Free summaries, full text may be available through a Lamaze membership or your local library.

Science and Sensibility Lamaze International publishes this regularly updated blog, and addresses many research related topics.

Understanding Research A site with links to many of the above resources, plus articles on how to find the studies you need, how to be a critical reader, and more. Also a glossary of research terms and links to many other resources.

State of the Worlds Midwifery National Governments Research Sites:

CDC, the US Census, and The Public Health Agency of Canada, These governmental agencies can be a trove of information on rates of births, deaths, conditions, etc. It may take a good chunk of time to mine through all the data, but there is useful information there.

World Health Organization It's not just for third world countries. The World Health Organization has lots of information on many aspects of maternal/child health. Check out the free downloadable publications.

Made in the USA
Monee, IL
06 August 2023

40528985R10136